CHANGING BEHAVIOR IN DBT

CHANGING BEHAVIOR in DBT

Problem Solving in Action

Heidi L. Heard
Michaela A. Swales

Foreword by Marsha M. Linehan

THE GUILFORD PRESS
New York   London

© 2016 The Guilford Press
A Division of Guilford Publications, Inc.
370 Seventh Avenue, Suite 1200, New York, NY 10001
www.guilford.com

Printed in the United States of America

This book is printed on acid-free paper.

Last digit is print number: 9 8 7 6 5 4 3 2

The authors have checked with sources believed to be reliable in their
efforts to provide information that is complete and generally in accord
with the standards of practice that are accepted at the time of publication.
However, in view of the possibility of human error or changes in behavioral,
mental health, or medical sciences, neither the authors, nor the editors and
publisher, nor any other party who has been involved in the preparation or
publication of this work warrants that the information contained herein is
in every respect accurate or complete, and they are not responsible for any
errors or omissions or the results obtained from the use of such information.
Readers are encouraged to confirm the information contained in this book
with other sources.

Library of Congress Cataloging-in-Publication Data

Names: Heard, Heidi L., author. | Swales, Michaela A., 1965– author.
Title: Changing behavior in DBT : problem solving in action / by Heidi L.
  Heard, Michaela A. Swales ; foreword by Marsha M. Linehan.
Description: New York : The Guilford Press, [2016] | Includes bibliographical
  references and index.
Identifiers: LCCN 2015034379 | ISBN 9781462522644 (hardback : acid-free paper)
Subjects: LCSH: Dialectical behavior therapy. | Behavior therapy. | BISAC:
  MEDICAL / Psychiatry / General. | SOCIAL SCIENCE / Social Work. |
  PSYCHOLOGY / Psychopathology / General.
Classification: LCC RC489.B4 H43 2016 | DDC 616.89/142—dc23
LC record available at http://lccn.loc.gov/2015034379

For those family and friends who provided
abundant support throughout this project
—H. L. H.

For Richard, Thomas, and Caitlin
—M. A. S.

ABOUT THE AUTHORS

Heidi L. Heard, PhD, has published numerous articles and chapters related to borderline personality disorder and DBT and is coauthor (with Michaela A. Swales) of *Dialectical Behaviour Therapy: Distinctive Features*. She collaborated with Dr. Marsha Linehan on the initial outcome trials for standard DBT and the adaptation for substance abuse and dependence, particularly focusing on the cost-effectiveness of DBT. Now retired, Dr. Heard was the founder of British Isles DBT Training and was a senior trainer for Behavioral Tech, which provides advanced training in DBT internationally. She provided consultation in the United States and Europe to DBT teams working in adult and adolescent outpatient programs and in adult secure inpatient programs, and to individual clinicians in adult outpatient, secure hospital, and prison settings.

Michaela A. Swales, PhD, is a Consultant Clinical Psychologist and Professor in Clinical Psychology on the North Wales Clinical Psychology Programme, Bangor University. She trained in DBT with Marsha Linehan and for 20 years ran a clinical program for suicidal young people in an inpatient service. Dr. Swales is Director of the British Isles DBT Training Team, an international affiliate of the Linehan Institute. She has trained more than a thousand professionals in DBT, seeding over 400 programs globally. She coauthored *Dialectical Behaviour Therapy: Distinctive Features* (with Heidi L. Heard) and is editor of the *Oxford Handbook of Dialectical Behaviour Therapy*. Her primary research interest is the effective implementation of evidence-based psychological therapies in routine clinical practice. Dr. Swales was a member of the Working Group on Classification of Personality Disorders reporting to the World Health Organization's International Advisory Group for the Revision of the ICD-10 Mental and Behavioural Disorders.

FOREWORD

Heidi Heard and Michaela Swales first met at one of my early intensive trainings in Seattle in the early 1990s. Heidi was then my graduate student; having been closely involved in the first randomized controlled trial of DBT, she was developing her skills as a trainer in DBT alongside me. Michaela was part of the first U.K. team to learn DBT. Inspired by her mentor, Mark Williams, who later went on to develop mindfulness-based cognitive therapy with John Teasdale and Zindel Segal, she had come to Seattle to learn how to treat adolescents with suicidal and self-harm behaviors. Heidi and Michaela's meeting was to prove auspicious for the dissemination of DBT outside the United States. They gave a presentation together at a conference in Dublin the following year, and during their visit there, they hatched the plan that would take Heidi to work alongside Michaela and Mark Williams in North Wales.

During Heidi's time in the United Kingdom, she used her already considerable skills and expertise to found the British Isles DBT Training Team, which Michaela would go on to lead. Together they have crossed the length and breadth of the United Kingdom and Ireland to train mental health professionals in DBT, eventually developing a national training team that delivers high-quality training in DBT throughout the British Isles, in partnership with the Linehan Institute. Their skills in mentoring trainers to achieve similar levels of precision and clarity in the conceptualization and treatment of clients' problems have informed the development of our own U.S. mentorship program for DBT trainers.

As well as being adherent and highly competent therapists themselves, Heidi and Michaela have developed a wealth and breadth of knowledge both in training therapists and developing their skills toward adherence to DBT, and in effectively implementing DBT in various health care systems. Their skills in training and consultation were recognized by the International Society for the Improvement of Training in DBT in 2009 with the Cindy Sanderson Outstanding Educator Award. This accolade came soon after the publication of their first book. *Dialectical Behaviour Therapy: Distinctive Features* provided an introductory overview of the treatment, helping those new to the therapy to develop a structural basis for more comprehensive learning of DBT.

This fabulous new book distills the knowledge Heidi and Michaela have gained in helping therapists learn and deliver the problem-solving component of DBT. Clients who come for treatment with DBT have complex and challenging problems. Their therapists have to work with them to change these previously intractable problems in a context of high risk and intense despair. Those therapists need this book. Precision and clarity in conceptual analysis and practical implementation are demonstrated on every page. In each chapter, Heidi and Michaela explicitly and succinctly highlight the principles of each step in problem solving in DBT. In their extensive experience, they have discerned the most common ways in which problem solving in DBT can go awry. Each of these common problems is described here with detailed illustrative case examples, and, crucially, Heidi and Michaela highlight how to resolve these issues in ways that promote the effectiveness of the treatment. Though what is written here is within the framework of DBT, therapists of many different cognitive-behavioral perspectives and persuasions will find much of practical relevance in this wonderful volume. Heidi and Michaela have written a book that will assist not only therapists new to DBT, but those more experienced as therapists or supervisors, in identifying and resolving typical problems in the execution of DBT—and thus improving clinical outcomes and the lives of our clients.

Readers are lucky to get a book by these two fabulous DBT therapists and trainers. This is particularly true when the topic is problem solving. We all know that this is often the significant challenge facing our clients: They cannot solve the major problems of their lives. But helping a client solve life problems isn't easy. This book by two therapists who know what they are doing is going to help you immensely.

MARSHA M. LINEHAN, PHD, ABPP
Professor and Director
Behavioral Research and Therapy Clinics
University of Washington

ACKNOWLEDGMENTS

When we first learned DBT we were struck by its compassion, optimism, and encouragement to persevere in changing the troubled lives of the people it seeks to treat. All of those things still hold true and, after 20 years of using the treatment, we continue to be amazed by its richness and flexibility in creatively deploying the principles of behavior change to address seemingly intractable problems. In treating patients in a myriad of different settings and training therapists in different cultures and settings, the principles initially described in Marsha M. Linehan's original manual have never let us down. As a result, our respect for Marsha's achievements in developing and testing the treatment has only increased. We wholeheartedly thank Marsha for the gift she gave us by training us in DBT and promoting our proficiency in its execution. We particularly want to thank her for contributing the foreword to this book.

We would like to express our sincerest gratitude to the delightful staff at The Guilford Press, who have been so supportive throughout the process. We especially want to thank Kitty Moore, who guided the book from its conception; Barbara Watkins, who provided significant suggestions on the manuscript; and Nina Hnatov, who copyedited the manuscript. When we received Kitty's feedback on the initial outline for the book, we were delighted to discover that we had an editor whom we could respect and trust. Over time we also learned that we had an editor who has extensive patience, infinite sympathy, and a sophisticated sense of humor. Barbara's feedback on the manuscript indicated that she had read every word from the first page through the last, one of the most validating things that any editor can do. We are eternally grateful for all of her corrections and comments, which will enhance the effectiveness of the book for readers. We are equally appreciative of Nina's copyediting. She caught our incidents of unmindful writing, corrected our errors, and minimized the likelihood that we would humiliate ourselves in public.

We wish to thank the many therapists whom we have trained and supervised over the years and who graciously accepted our feedback and shaping, frequently within the public setting of DBT intensive trainings. Over years of teaching DBT, we have observed that therapists, often working in systems with limited access to supervision, make similar errors when trying to help clients change behavior. We hope that this book encapsulates these problems and elucidates some solutions in ways that will promote DBT therapists' adherence and competence and ultimately improve the lives of their clients. To accomplish this, we have tried to model a rigorous application of principles, rather than a rigid application of rules. We anticipate that if therapists mindfully apply these principles and related strategies, they will be rewarded with mastery in analyzing problems, creating solutions, and changing behaviors.

—Heidi L. Heard and Michaela A. Swales

There are innumerable contributors to this book. It would not exist without the inspiration provided by supervisees and trainees who have asked stimulating questions, sought consultation on their formulations and therapy-session recordings, and collaboratively role-played during our sessions. Similarly, I appreciate how much clients have taught me and particularly thank them for tolerating how much I needed to learn. I also want to acknowledge the contribution of those DBT colleagues who have helped me over the years by modeling problem solving, generously sharing clinical examples and teaching stories, and providing me with constructive feedback on my teaching and writing. Finally, I especially want to thank Michaela for her collaboration, tolerance, and loyalty throughout our long partnership.

—Heidi L. Heard

My greatest thanks go to my husband, Richard, and my children, Caitlin and Thomas. Without their continuous support and willingness to do without me, I would never have been able to put in the therapy and training hours to develop the skills and knowledge upon which this book is based, much less find the time to write it! I also wish to thank my professional colleagues within DBT whose own skills, knowledge, and enthusiasm have contributed in no small way to what you see written here. At the head of this queue is my coauthor, Heidi Heard, who has been my constant companion on the journey of learning, delivering, and teaching DBT. Her friendship and conceptual rigor have been the two most consistent features of my professional life. Thanks also to Christine Dunkley and Janet Feigenbaum, two inspirational clinicians who have aided and abetted Heidi and me in disseminating DBT across the United Kingdom and Ireland. Without the support and facilitative style of my employer, Betsi Cadwaladr University Health Board, and the School of Psychology, Bangor University, none of my achievements in DBT would have been possible. Special thanks to Robin Glaze and Colin Elliott, who, in different ways, exercised tolerance and flexibility around the demands that training others in DBT placed on my other work roles.

—*Michaela A. Swales*

CONTENTS

CHAPTER 1

CHANGING BEHAVIOR IN DBT

An Overview

Just hours after your therapy appointment with an outpatient client, the emergency room phones to inform you that the client has taken a nearly lethal overdose. You wonder what led to this overdose. Was it your refusal to extend the therapy session, and was the client still angry with you? Is that why she overdosed instead of phoning for coaching? During the session, she spoke about an argument with her boyfriend earlier in the day and described worries and fear that he would leave her. Did she have another argument with him or did he leave her? Was the overdose a suicide attempt and what was its function? Was she trying to express anger toward you, to convince her boyfriend that she needed him or to reduce her fear of being alone? Shame, warranted and unwarranted, has often precipitated her suicide attempts; could it have played a role in this overdose? How will you analyze which variables caused the overdose and then effectively treat those variables to reduce the likelihood of another overdose? Will you contact her in the hospital to strengthen your relationship or just expect her for your next scheduled appointment? If not extending the last session was a causal link to the overdose, will you give her more time in the future or will you teach her other ways to manage her anger? If warranted shame led to the overdose, will you try to soothe away her shame or encourage her to implement a repair? If an argument with her boyfriend led to the overdose, does she need to learn interpersonal skills or does anger toward the boyfriend interfere with her interpersonal skills? Do they need couple therapy to change the way he responds to her overdoses? Does

1

she need to challenge her worry thoughts about him leaving her or should she leave him?

A day before your scheduled appointment with an inpatient client, the patient's psychiatrist informs you that the patient has threatened to report you for "bullying." You assume that the patient must be angry with you but do not know what prompted this threat and do not know the function of the behavior. Will you contact the patient as soon as possible to repair the relationship or will you wait until the scheduled appointment to address the threat? When asked for examples of "bullying" the patient gives examples of dialectical behavior therapy confrontation and solution implementation strategies (which your supervisor has approved as adherent). Should you stop using these strategies to avoid the complaint, challenge the patient's accusation of bullying, or help the patient to write the complaint as skillfully as possible?

Therapists providing dialectical behavior therapy (DBT; Linehan, 1993a) answer the questions raised by clients' clinical behaviors by applying a complex set of principles. When a DBT therapist targets a specific clinical behavior for change (e.g., overdoses, threatening therapists, bingeing and purging), the most directly relevant and important principles are those that allow the therapist to develop a behavioral conceptualization and to decide which problem-solving strategies to implement and how to implement them. Though several DBT books address these principles and practices to some extent, this book is the first devoted to the topic. The book uses two decades of experience since the first publication of Linehan's books (1993a, 1993b) to illustrate these key principles and practices and to resolve common problems relevant to targeting clinical behaviors.

In this book, we first aim to highlight and clarify the key principles used in the development of behavioral conceptualizations and the selection of problem-solving strategies. The book particularly emphasizes the importance of conceptual clarity. It also attends to the adherent application of the most relevant problem-solving strategies, though it does not attempt to review all of these strategies, as Linehan's treatment manual (1993a) has already accomplished this task.

Though the principles and practices have not changed substantially since the treatment manual's initial publication, the last two decades have increased the awareness of the many challenges that therapists repeatedly encounter and of the mistakes they may make when trying to apply the behavioral aspects of the treatment. For example, a therapist conducting a chain analysis of a targeted behavior may become "lost" if he or she poorly defined the behavior or the client repeatedly returns to describing a narrative of his or her week. Alternatively, the analysis may stall if the client repeatedly responds with "I can't remember." Such problems will increase further if the therapist then inadvertently reinforces the client's behaviors, for example, by listening attentively to a narrative of the client's week or automatically stopping the analysis if the client "can't remember." A therapist and client might have generated a variety of conceptually appropriate solutions to match a chain analysis, but the client might then refuse to implement any of the solutions. Alternatively, the therapist might believe that the solutions are being implemented in the session when the therapist and client actually are only further discussing them. In this book, we also aim to identify common problems such as these and to suggest effective ways to minimize mistakes and resolve challenges.

Since the publication of Linehan's (1993a, 1993b) books, the application of DBT has extended beyond the original target population of suicidal clients with borderline personality disorder (BPD). Although this book focuses primarily on clients who meet criteria for BPD, clinical examples include a variety of target behaviors, not just suicidal behaviors. Examples also derive from incarcerated, forensic clients (e.g., forensic hospitals) with antisocial personality disorder as an important diagnosis, and from adolescent clients, some in traditional DBT and some in the adolescent adaptation (Miller, Rathus, & Linehan, 2006), who do not yet meet criteria for any personality disorder. Though the book has the most relevance for DBT individual therapy, it includes a few examples from other DBT treatment modalities, especially the consultation team. As ethics and custom dictate, we have created composite clinical vignettes, based on our experiences of delivering the treatment and training therapists over the last two decades. We have purposefully selected scenarios that represent common experiences or typical problems to maximize the generalizability of the example, while avoiding the identification of a specific person. No clinical vignette describes an actual client or therapist, thus any resemblance to a specific person is purely coincidental.

AN OVERVIEW OF THE BOOK

The remainder of this chapter describes the broader DBT context in which therapists develop behavioral conceptualizations and implement problem-solving strategies. Standard behavior theories and a biosocial theory, developed to explain the behaviors associated with BPD, provide the theoretical context for the treatment and the key principles used in behavioral formulations. DBT also attends to dialectical principles, which describe how progress, or at least change, occurs through a process of opposition and synthesis. To achieve synthesis and progress, the treatment incorporates practices of acceptance to balance behavioral problem solving, a practice of change. In addition to reviewing the relevant theoretical principles, this first chapter describes how a behavioral approach impacts some of the structural elements of the treatment and how other therapy strategies balance or enhance the problem-solving strategies.

The subsequent chapters each illustrate the key concepts and strategies of behavioral problem solving and discuss common challenges and errors in their application. Chapter 2 attends to the development and implementation of a DBT target hierarchy of problem behaviors to be treated. The primary components of problem solving are divided into behavioral chain analysis (BCA), covered in Chapter 3, and solution analysis, covered in Chapter 4. The chain analysis functions to help the therapist and client to identify the controlling variables of a targeted behavior and consequently to obtain the information needed for an effective solution analysis. The solution analysis functions to help the therapist and client to identify and implement the most effective cognitive-behavioral therapy (CBT) procedures to change the controlling variables and consequently change the target behavior.

Each of the remaining chapters presents the CBT procedures utilized as solutions in DBT. Chapter 5 addresses the skills training component of the therapy. It discusses aspects common to teaching clients any skill, namely skills acquisition, strengthening, and generalization, as opposed to reviewing each specific DBT skill set. Chapters 6, 7, and 8 all focus on treating motivational variables that control the targeted behavior. Chapter 6 discusses the treatment of classically conditioned responses and includes sections on both stimulus control and exposure. Chapter 7 considers the treatment of cognitive behaviors, with particular attention to how a behavioral treatment of cognitive processes differs from cognitive treatment. Chapter 8 discusses the treatment of operant responses and the implementation of contingency management.

Clarifying Terms

At this point, it may prove useful to clarify several terms used throughout the book. First, DBT emphasizes the use of "principles." The following best defines the use of the term in this book: "a general truth, a law comprehending many sub-ordinate truths, . . . the primary source from which anything proceeds, a basic doctrine or tenet, . . . a law on which others are founded or from which others are derived" (Webster's New Collegiate Dictionary, 1981, p. 757). Though all therapies derive from a theory and corresponding set of principles, they differ in how much they attend to and rely on these principles in each session. Therapies also differ in the extent to which they rely on general principles or develop specific protocols. In DBT, the principles deserve attention throughout the session. They remain at a relatively general level, however, in contrast to more traditional forms of CBT that have specific protocols for each session. (One could describe a protocol for a DBT session as briefly as select a behavior to target, conduct a BCA, and apply a solution analysis.) This close attention to general principles enables therapists to apply the treatment both rigorously to enhance adherence to the model and flexibly to enhance responsiveness to the client. Unfortunately, learning to apply treatment models that depend on principles can prove challenging. Therapists, like most humans, often prefer to know the protocols and follow them automatically rather than having to decide which principle to apply, how to apply it, and what to do if two principles conflict with each other. The protocols usually prove easier and often *seem* safer; unfortunately, they often prove less effective.

This book uses the term "behavioral conceptualization," or formulation, as a distinct term that differs from the more common meaning of case conceptualization or formulation. As commonly used, case conceptualization refers to a broad overview of a client's clinical problems (e.g., diagnoses and presenting problems), a history and explanation of the cause of those problems (often including distant historical factors), and a summary of the longer-term treatment plan. Therapists create such case conceptualizations at the beginning of therapy, and these conceptualizations generally evolve slowly over time. In contrast, this book uses "behavioral conceptualization" to refer to a much more specific understanding of the immediate factors that control an instance of a targeted behavior. Each targeted episode of a behavior has its own behavioral formulation, though one formulation may influence the next if the targeted behaviors or their contexts resemble each other. The behavioral formulation provides a specific definition of the problem behavior, analyzes the most proximate factors controlling the behavior, and develops a detailed treatment plan designed for immediate implementation.

As the book attends extensively to the common problems in applying key principles and practices, it might also prove useful to consider the parameters of included problems. All of the errors and issues described here have occurred in either teaching or supervising on multiple occasions. The book includes errors that could cause enduring harm to a client, but fortunately relatively few errors have this impact. Many of the included problems, however, increase some type of distress during the session. For example, making assumptions about the function of the client's behavior rather than generating hypotheses increases the likelihood of invalidating the client. Many problems decrease the efficacy or efficiency of either a session or even the course of treatment. For example, suggesting new skills without practicing them in the session tends to decrease the likelihood that the client will use the skill outside of the session or use it effectively. Waiting for insight to emerge from the client rather than using mind reading or hypothesis testing tends only to prolong the chain analysis and consequently preempt the solution analysis. The book includes problems that reduce the therapist's adherence, the therapist's motivation to apply the treatment, and the client's motivation to participate in the treatment. Though each chapter includes a distinct section for the identification and discussion of these common problems, potential problems may also appear in the sections describing key principles if the problem flows directly from not applying the principle.

Though aware of the debate regarding the terminology used to denote the person receiving a psychological treatment, we have chosen simply to utilize the most common appellation for each relevant setting, namely "client" for a person treated in the community and "patient" for a person treated on an inpatient unit. As the individual therapy modality of DBT meets the criteria for a psychotherapy, as defined by Corsini and Wedding (1989), we could utilize the term "psychotherapist" to denote professionals delivering this modality. Linehan (1993a), however, chose the more generic term "therapist" for her treatment manual, and we continue this tradition. Of course, "skills trainers" refers to professionals leading a skills training group or conducting scheduled skills training sessions with an individual client. "Skills coach" refers to a professional with the assigned role of helping clients to generalize DBT skills, for example, through telephone coaching with outpatients or ad hoc in-person coaching on an inpatient unit.

DBT FOUNDATIONS FOR BEHAVIORAL CHANGE

DBT is a behavioral therapy founded on principles from learning theory and problem-solving therapies. It synthesizes these principles with principles from dialectics and Zen Buddhism. We next discuss these foundations for DBT and how DBT adapts them.

Learning Theory

Behavioral learning theories and the family of therapies that derive from them underlie the process of changing behavior with DBT. Learning theories incorporated in DBT include classical conditioning and operant conditioning, as well as Staats's (1975) unified theory of social or psychological behaviorism. These learning theories inform the theoretical basis of the treatment, describing how the emotional and behavioral problems initially develop and, more importantly, how these problems are maintained in the present. Much of this learning occurs out of the client's awareness, and thus without the client's intent. These theories both contribute to therapists' broad case conceptualizations of clients' problems and directly inform the specific behavioral conceptualization that therapists develop within each session. Therapists use the theories to identify controlling variables for clients' behaviors and to generate related solutions. This section provides a brief overview of some of the key terms and concepts of these theories.

Classical Conditioning

Classical conditioning, identified first by Pavlov (1927), describes a process through which an animal learns or changes a response to a stimulus through the pairing of that stimulus with another stimulus and its natural response. Building on his observations of the biological reflex response that dogs salivate (unconditioned response) when presented with food (unconditioned stimulus), Pavlov next observed that when the sound of a bell (conditioned stimulus) was repeatedly paired with the presentation of food (unconditioned stimulus), dogs learned to salivate (unconditioned response) to the sound of the bell alone. His research then influenced approaches to behavioral case formulation that saw the role of respondent or classical conditioning in the development of human psychopathology. Most famously perhaps, Watson (Watson & Rayner, 1920) taught little Albert to fear rats. Initially, the infant Albert had a natural, unconditioned fear response to loud noises but not to rats. The researchers then simultaneously produced the loud noise (unconditioned stimulus) and presented the rat (conditioned stimulus). After several trials, poor Albert exhibited a learned, conditioned fear response to the rat alone. This pattern of learning responses underpins the behavioral conceptualization of a number of anxiety-based responses, for example, in phobias, obsessive–compulsive disorders, and posttraumatic stress disorder.

With an understanding of how classical conditioning contributes to some types of dysfunctional responses, researchers began to experiment with ways to apply the same conditioning processes to the treatment of those responses. Mary Cover Jones (1924) pioneered the use of classical conditioning processes to treat phobias when she successfully treated little Peter's fear of rabbits by pairing the presentation of food (unconditioned stimulus), which elicited pleasure (unconditioned response), and a rabbit (conditioned stimulus), which elicited fear (a dysfunctional conditioned response). Decades later, Wolpe (1958) developed the highly successful and widely used procedure of systematic desensitization by devising hierarchies of fear-producing stimuli that he systematically presented to his clients while the client practiced deep-muscle relaxation. Subsequent research has revealed that successful treatment requires neither the hierarchy nor the deep-muscle relaxation, but does require exposure to relevant stimuli.

CLASSICAL CONDITIONING IN DBT

DBT therapists' focus on identifying conditioned stimuli and responses among the antecedents of target behaviors owes much to the work of Jones, Wolpe, and their successors. For example, during the early stages of therapy a DBT therapist noticed that her client had an aversive response to praise: the client visibly shrank back from the therapist, started to shake, and typically decreased her skillful behavior. When the therapist inquired about these responses, the client reported experiencing anxiety and thinking that the therapist was about to discharge her whenever the therapist praised her. The therapist knew that the client had experienced many different psychological treatments and interventions from her local mental health team over the years. Generally these interventions began during crises, continued for several months, and terminated when the client ceased her suicidal behavior. On withdrawal of services the client gradually became more anxious and coped less well, eventually returning to suicidal behavior. The therapist hypothesized that the client's history of repeated pairings of praise about progress (conditioned stimulus) with discussions about withdrawal of services (unconditioned stimulus) resulted in the anxiety, which was originally an unconditioned response to withdrawal of services, becoming a conditioned response to praise. The therapist also noticed that the conditioned anxiety had generalized to other stimuli, such as the therapist speaking in an upbeat tone of voice. The therapist's nonverbal behavior signaled to the client that praise may soon occur, though the client had no awareness of this learned response. As therapy progressed the therapist repeatedly presented cues about progress, delivered in an upbeat tone, and then returned to working together on solving the client's problems. This approach presented the client with a new pairing, praise linked to continued discussion of problems, which gradually reduced the client's conditioned anxiety to praise. Chapter 6 discusses exposure and related solutions in detail.

Operant Conditioning

Operant conditioning describes the processes whereby animals learn to associate a behavior with specific consequences and those consequences of the behavior then significantly control the probability of that behavior reoccurring. Skinner (1953, 1976) used the term "operant" as he viewed many behaviors as "operating" on the environment in ways that produced certain consequences. A contingent relationship thus exists between the operant behavior and its consequences. Consistent with many forms of behavior therapy, DBT therapists use behavioral analyses to assess and describe the contingent relationships related to target behaviors. Therapists and clients can then apply contingency management (see Chapter 8) to change problematic contingent relationships.

Operant conditioning includes the processes of reinforcement and punishment. These processes contribute both to the development and maintenance of clients' problematic behaviors. Reinforcement occurs when a consequence of a behavior increases the likelihood that the behavior will occur again. Most clients identify the removal of aversive affects as the type of consequence that primarily reinforces suicidal and many other target behaviors. Sometimes, however, one consequence alone initially reinforces a behavior, but as additional consequences occur they too become reinforcing. For example, one client had a long history of reducing her anxiety with overdoses. When her husband spent time away with his friends, she would become anxious about coping alone and would overdose to decrease her anxiety. Feeling guilty, her husband would then spend more time with her. This increased time with her husband also became a reinforcer for overdosing. In addition to considering multiple reinforcing consequences, the therapist must differentiate reinforcing consequences from neutral consequences. For example, attempting suicide may lead to a decrease in emotions, an ambulance ride, care from psychiatric staff, and reduced domestic responsibilities. The care from staff would reinforce the attempt among some clients, the reduction of domestic responsibilities would do so among others, and some clients would be reinforced by both or neither. At least one client's suicidal behavior increased as a consequence of the arousal associated with ambulance rides.

Positive reinforcement occurs when the consequence involves the addition of pleasurable stimuli or a reward, whereas negative reinforcement occurs when the consequence includes the subtraction or removal of aversive stimuli. Examples of consequences that negatively reinforce suicide attempts, substance abuse, bulimia, and other impulsive behaviors include a decrease in bodily tension, removal of unwanted emotions, and relief from distressing thoughts. Examples of consequences that cause positive reinforcement include gaining a sense of control, validation of self-constructs, and more care or support from the environment.

Punishment, in contrast, occurs when a consequence to a behavior results on average in a decrease in that behavior. For example, many clients report that whenever they expressed negative emotions during childhood, their families responded with ridicule, physical isolation, or physical punishment. These consequences commonly punished the emotional expression, teaching clients to inhibit instead. The common practice of ending treatment interventions as soon as a crisis behavior ends can punish coping behaviors in clients who need or want longer-term treatment. Positive punishment occurs when the consequence adds aversive stimuli, whereas negative punishment occurs when the consequence includes the subtraction or removal of pleasurable stimuli. One client experienced both types of punishment when trying to develop more skillful and functional behavior. First, when she made a commitment to stop cutting herself, she gave her self-harm paraphernalia to her therapist as a sign of her commitment. She immediately experienced increasing anxiety and more frequent suicidal thoughts and decreased her willingness to commit to implementing other solutions. In this case, the *addition* of undesirable consequences—namely, increased anxiety and suicidal thinking—led to the positive punishment of her skillful behavior of committing to solutions. Later in therapy this client began to spend an increasing amount of time working. Her husband then announced that now that she was more financially secure he could leave her for another woman; her work hours quickly decreased. In these circumstances, the *removal* of something desirable to her—namely, her relationship with her husband—negatively punished her for working to support herself financially.

Problem Solving

Problem solving as a therapeutic approach has a well-established history within the CBTs since the seminal work of D'Zurilla and Goldfried

(1971). Treatment developers have applied the approach to a variety of psychiatric problems ranging from depression (Nezu, Nezu, & Perri, 1989) to schizophrenia (Falloon, Boyd, & McGill, 1984). A review (Heard, 2002) of psychosocial treatment studies for suicidal and non-suicidal self-injurious behaviors noted the relative effectiveness of problem-solving therapy (e.g., McLeavey, Daly, Ludgate, & Murray, 1994; Salkovskis, Atha, & Storer, 1990; Van der Sande et al., 1997), though the review also highlighted that most of the problem-solving conditions modified standard outpatient therapy to include either intensive care (e.g., brief planned hospitalizations) or outreach care (e.g., home visits, telephone contact).

Problem-solving therapies postulate that maladaptive behavior occurs when individuals lack the psychological resources to resolve their problems in any other way. To help clients develop the necessary resources to change the maladaptive behavior, problem-solving therapies (e.g., D'Zurilla & Nezu, 1999; Hawton & Kirk, 1989) teach clients a systematic method for solving current as well as any future personal problems. The therapy begins by clearly defining a client's problems and helping the client to establish realistic goals. For example, a relatively vague problem like "I don't get along with people" becomes "I criticize family members so much that they say they don't want to spend time with me." Once the client has sufficiently described the problem, the therapist and client together creatively generate or "brainstorm" possible solutions. For example, the "critical" client could stop criticizing completely, more selectively choose what and whom he or she criticizes, use interpersonal skills to criticize more effectively, balance criticism with praise, or learn to decrease unwarranted critical thinking. The therapist and client then consider the possible outcomes for these solutions. For example, to stop criticizing completely could mean that the client would endure others' behaviors that actually harmed the client's welfare. After the therapist and client have chosen the most viable solutions, the client tries them, both in and out of session. As part of this process, the therapist might apply a number of CBT procedures, including cognitive modification, role plays of interpersonal skills, contingency management, and didactics. Finally, the therapist and client review the effectiveness of the solutions and modify them accordingly. For example, the client might have chosen to validate the other person before saying something critical, but when the client rehearses this in the session, the therapist quickly realizes that the client's attempt at validation sounds more like sarcasm. The therapist would then need to solve that problem with the solution or try another solution.

In addition to the specific strategies of the approach, problem-solving therapies adhere to the general principles and practices of CBTs. At the beginning of therapy, the therapist and client agree on therapeutic goals and a time frame for the therapy. During the course of therapy, the therapist focuses primarily on the "here and now," emphasizes learning that leads directly to change in daily life, and explicitly explains theory and techniques to the client. With regard to assessing treatment efficacy and effectiveness, these therapies apply an objective, scientific approach to both a specific client and a particular client population alike.

DBT Adaptations of Problem-Solving Therapies

Although DBT implements the basic practices and principles of behavior therapy in general and problem-solving therapy in particular, it has also adapted or added to the theory, structure, and strategies of the traditional therapy approach to address the challenges of treating complex clients who have a personality disorder diagnosis. The addition of dialectical and Zen principles and a biosocial theory of BPD are discussed later in this chapter. Changes to the structure of standard problem-solving therapies generally reflect the client populations of most DBT programs, namely severe, chronic, multidiagnostic populations that have not succeeded in other standard treatments. In contrast to traditional problem-solving therapies that have historically lasted for 3 months or less, most outpatient DBT programs require an initial 1-year commitment from clients. This time frame accommodates the slower progress of severe clients, allows time to address the multiple problems of multidiagnostic clients, and mitigates against the "revolving-door" experience of chronic clients. Comprehensive DBT programs, inpatient and outpatient alike, also offer multiple but *integrated* treatment modalities concurrently, similar to the way that problem-solving therapies for suicide often added outreach or intensity to their treatment. In addition to doing problem solving in individual therapy sessions, clients attend a group that teaches them a package of skills to try as solutions, and they can access skills coaching between sessions. Though each component serves a specific function, together they increase the frequency of DBT as a stimulus that can prompt and reinforce adaptive behaviors. Sharing a client with someone on the same treatment team who works within the same conceptual frame may also help to reduce the common stressful experiences (e.g., anxiety, frustration, and confusion) that therapists have when working with these clients. Finally, DBT programs use a structured target hierarchy as part of the case conceptualization to determine the order in which therapists will treat clients' problem behaviors. Such target hierarchies decrease the likelihood of therapists being overwhelmed by the multiple diagnoses and other problems experienced by most clients with BPD and increase the likelihood that therapists will progress methodically in treating the most severe problems rather than respond reactively by treating the crisis of the week.

In standard DBT programs, the target hierarchy focuses on (1) suicidal, homicidal, and other imminently life-threatening behaviors; (2) therapy-interfering behaviors (TIBs) by either the therapist or client; and (3) "quality-of-life-interfering" behaviors. "Quality-of-life-interfering" behaviors include specific criteria of psychiatric disorders (e.g., bingeing and purging for bulimia nervosa, compulsive cleaning for obsessive–compulsive disorder) and severe behaviors that cause substantial instability (e.g., arguing with roommates that leads to homelessness, impulsive spending that leads to unmanageable debt) or require intervention by others (e.g., child neglect requiring social services involvement, illegal activity requiring police involvement, problematic employment behavior leading to living on welfare). See Chapter 2 for more on targeting.

To traditional problem-solving strategies, Linehan (1993a) has added the use of behavioral chain analyses to obtain more detailed information about the causal links leading to and following from a specific episode of a target behavior. Chapter 3 describes this set of strategies in detail. The addition of a chain analysis helps the therapist and client to cope with the complexity of the client's problems by focusing their attention on identifying the most important controlling variables (e.g., prompting event, cognitions, affect, impulses, and consequences) of a specific episode of a specific targeted behavior. They do not need to concern themselves with stories of all of the similar episodes of behavior nor with all of the other experiences of the day. At the same time, a chain analysis prevents them from oversimplifying the complexity of the problem by attending to only one aspect of the problem. For example, if a therapist asked a new client, "Why did you harm yourself?" the client might simply respond with "My boyfriend was a jerk" and fail to identify important links that a chain analysis would identify, such as judgments of him, ruminating on his past behavior, anger toward him, the thought "I'll show him," and his apologies when he learns what she has done "because of him."

Finally, although behavior therapies regularly attend to the therapy relationship (Gilbert & Leahy, 2007; Meichenbaum & Turk, 1987), DBT attends more closely than most. As many of these clients have a history of failed therapy relationships, DBT therapists attempt to identify potential problems at the earliest stage possible and then track and directly treat these problems as they occur. DBT therapists, however, do not consider these problems only as obstacles to avoid or overcome so that the "real" therapy can proceed. Instead, the therapist treats them as examples of the relationship problems that occur in the rest of the client's life and as the most immediate opportunities to learn problem solving. For example, a client who refuses to phone his or her therapist for skills coaching because he or she is still mad at the therapist for not extending the session may also refuse to talk with family or friends following conflict with them. By treating the most important links leading to the TIB (e.g., judgments about and intense anger toward the therapist, then shame about being so angry, followed by the urge to hide away), the client may also learn how to respond more effectively after conflict with family and friends. As discussed in Chapter 8, if a client generally values the therapeutic relationship, then the therapist can also use elements of the relationship to motivate the client.

Dialectical Principles

Based originally on a set of practices intended to search for truth through rational disagreement, dialectics evolved into a set of principles that aim to describe the nature of reality. Though dialectics derives from philosophical (e.g., Plato, 1969; Tucker, 1978, for Marx and Engels) rather than empirical origins, the application of dialectics now encompasses areas directly relevant to psychological treatments. Linehan's (1993a; Linehan & Schmidt, 1995) application of dialectics was influenced by evolutionary biology (Levins & Lewontin, 1985), cognitive development (Basseches, 1984), and the evolution of self (Kegan, 1982).

Dialectics suggests several assumptions about the nature of reality that have particular relevance to treating clients with BPD. First, reality is in a process of continuous change, and everything is transient. Thus, an individual's behaviors will change, for better or worse, and regardless of whether the individual receives treatment or not. The role of treatment is to direct and promote change along the most effective path toward a client's long-term goals.

Just as the client's behavior will naturally change over time, so too will elements in the environment, including relationships. For example, as the therapeutic relationship develops over time, the therapist may become willing to therapeutically expand various limits (e.g., strategical use of self-disclosure, availability for telephone consultation) as one would expand limits in any other relationship over time. Such limits could contract as well if the therapist's life changes (e.g., therapist has a baby or illness in the family) or the therapeutic relationship changes (e.g., client persistently phones too often). The therapist does not try to protect the client from such natural change but instead teaches the client how to cope with the change.

Dialectics proposes that change occurs as a consequence of opposing forces within a system transcending the tension and resolving into a synthesis that again evolves into a new tension. This proposal is based on the principles that everything contains opposing forces and that everything is interrelated. Levins and Lewontin (1985) describe the process of change: "Parts and wholes evolve in consequence of their relationship, and the relationship itself evolves" (p. 3). Dialectics thus contrasts with dualistic and reductionistic philosophies of science, the latter of which has been used by critics to describe behaviorism (Skinner, 1976).

The principle of interrelatedness highlights the transactional development of reality. In transactional development, two elements do not simply combine to create something new, they also shape each other during the process. Thus, in Linehan's (1993a) biosocial theory of BPD, the individual's biological temperament doesn't simply combine with an invalidating environment and consequently create BPD. The individual's temperament can actually shape the environment into becoming more invalidating, whereas an abusive, invalidating environment can have a permanent impact on temperament. Similarly, DBT therapists attend vigilantly to transactions that occur within the therapeutic context, a system in which the therapist and client reciprocally influence each other. The addition of a consultation team for therapists functions to increase the likelihood that the reciprocal influence leads to a reduction in clients' problems, rather than an increase in therapists' problems.

The principle of interrelatedness encourages a systemic approach to problem solving, both in terms of the conceptualization and the strategies. Regarding the behavioral conceptualization, DBT therapists assess for both internal and external factors that control behaviors, including biochemistry, information processing, affect, impulses, interpersonal responses, and culture. Therapists analyze the cause and-effect relationship among these factors from a transactional perspective that highlights how the factors reciprocally influence one another and that a causal factor in one moment may become an effect in the next moment. For example, Anna suffered from a serotonin imbalance that increased the likelihood of depressed moods. When depressed, she had difficulty solving problems in general and interpersonal problems in particular. She coped by withdrawing from her family. The withdrawal further increased cognitive impairment in the form of rumination. The withdrawal also elicited criticism from the family that prompted increased self-invalidation that exacerbated the depression. With impaired problem solving, Anna decided to solve the problem of the depression and criticism with an overdose. Hospitalized for the overdose, she received more validation from staff than she ever received from her family. A systemic approach also foresees how any single intervention may influence multiple systems. For example, pharmacotherapy may regulate serotonin intake such that the chain described above never begins. Alternatively, enhancing emotion regulation skills may help Anna to cope effectively with biological changes such that problem solving is not impaired. Managing contingencies of overdosing may diminish the likelihood that hospitalization reinforces any overdoses. With respect to problem-solving strategies, dialectics underlines the importance of attending to the interdependence of mechanisms of change. A client's tolerance for problem-solving strategies, for example, depends partly on interweaving them with validation strategies. The success of behavioral chain and solution analyses generally depend on their integration. Chain analyses alone may provide only insight, which usually proves insufficient for change, and requires the client to review the painful past without providing alternatives for the future. Solution analyses alone, however, risk invalidating the client and increase the likelihood of generating invalid solutions.

With respect to the principle that everything contains opposing forces, Linehan (1993a) identifies the central opposition in DBT as the tension between change and acceptance. CBT provides the foundation for change, while Zen principles, described more extensively below, provide the primary foundation for acceptance. DBT also synthesizes the change strategies of problem solving with the acceptance strategies of validation. The therapy strives to help the client understand that certain behaviors may prove both valid and problematic. For example, Diana feared not having sufficient skills to cope while her therapist went on vacation, and she began to threaten suicide. As she actually had few coping skills and functioned better when meeting her therapist weekly, her fear had validity. As threatening suicide had previously caused others to change their behavior in a way that decreased her distress, threatening had validity. Equally, the suicide threats caused problems as they increased the likelihood of a suicide attempt and decreased the therapist's motivation to treat Diana. The therapist synthesized problem solving and validation by offering an extra session prior to the vacation (after Diana committed to no suicide attempts), and then used the session to focus exclusively on skills to help Diana cope with the separation.

In therapy, tensions frequently arise between the client and therapist. Consistent with dialectics, DBT therapists view these tensions as opportunities rather than obstacles. To resolve these conflicts, therapists search for syntheses, with the most effective syntheses generally being those that validate both positions and refocus on a shared goal. For example, Daniel viewed his drug use as a solution, particularly to his chronic anxiety, while his therapist viewed the drug use as a problem, in itself and because it contributed to antisocial behaviors. They achieved a synthesis by identifying anxiety reduction as a valid therapy goal. With this as the mutual goal, the drug use lost some of its validity, as it actually maintained the long-term anxiety, despite providing short-term relief. The therapy then emphasized stimulus control, exposure, emotion regulation skills, and distress-tolerance skills to prevent or manage anxiety. When therapy does not successfully resolve tensions, TIBs often occur. For example, if his therapist simply confronted Daniel about the drug use but never offered alternative solutions for the anxiety, Daniel might have begun to lie about drug use. Therapists then treat these behaviors (the therapist's and client's alike) with the same behavioral conceptualization and problem-solving strategies as other target behaviors.

Principles from Zen

To balance the change focus of behaviorism, Linehan integrated into DBT principles and techniques from acceptance-based practices, especially from Zen. Her attention to acceptance and particularly to the Zen practice of mindfulness placed DBT among the vanguard of a new era of CBT approaches. She did not discuss the wider influence of Zen on the treatment in the original treatment manual, but has addressed these influences in other writings (e.g., Heard & Linehan, 2005). Zen principles about the nature of reality influence the treatment as a whole, including how therapists approach problem solving. In her most recent work, Linehan (2014) has elaborated on the spiritual origins of mindfulness skills from religious traditions other than Zen, assisting clients with religious faiths to engage with the practice. Though a thorough discussion of Zen principles is beyond the scope of this book, we highlight a few principles with particular relevance to the book.

Like behaviorism, Zen attempts to describe aspects of reality, including observations about causal relationships, learning, and development. The principle that the universe accepts all things as they are is consistent with behaviorists' nonjudgmental assessment of factors controlling behavior. Zen emphasizes "acceptance" at its most radical level.

The principle that "the essential world of perfection is this very world" (Aitken, 1982, p. 63) expresses the essence of acceptance in Zen. The world is "perfect" and "should" (in the conditional, not the judgmental meaning) be as it is; it cannot be any different than it is because it is created or caused by what has preceded it and that cannot be changed. For example, Diana, the client with the soon-to-vacation therapist, "should" feel anxious if she does not have the skills to cope as well during the separation. She "should" even threaten self-harm in response to the planned vacation if she has "intolerable" anxiety about it, and past learning has taught her that threatening suicide increases the likelihood that the other person will act in a way that reduces her anxiety.

Not accepting reality exacerbates existing problems or creates new ones. In his description of Zen, Aitken (1982, p. 49) comments on the inherent nature of suffering and the effects of not accepting it: "The first truth enunciated by the Buddha is that life is suffering. Avoidance of suffering leads to worse suffering. . . . We drink alcohol excessively to avoid that pain, thus causing more pain." Zen suggests that suffering results primarily from insatiable desires for or attachments to reality being a certain way. These desires or attachments have many forms, ranging from attachment to a set of beliefs to yearning for a particular relationship. For example, if the vacationing therapist remains attached to the belief that Diana should not threaten suicide and just ignores the behavior without first trying to understand it, the therapist may miss an opportunity for helping Diana to develop or may even lead Diana to escalate to an actual suicide attempt. Meanwhile, if Diana continues to threaten suicide to keep the therapist in town, the therapist may eventually decide to stop treating Diana altogether. When reality crashes into desire, the one with the driving desire receives the damage. Zen does not state that attachments or desire should not occur; it simply highlights their relationship to suffering and encourages letting go of them.

The impact of attachment has particular relevance for therapists learning a new therapy. The following story illustrates how attachments can interfere with learning:

> Nan-in, a Japanese master during the Meiji era (1868–1912), received a university professor who came to inquire about Zen. Nan-in served tea. He poured his visitor's cup full, and then kept on pouring.
>
> The professor watched the overflow until he no longer could restrain himself. "It is overfull. No more will go in!"
>
> "Like this cup," Nan-in said, "you are full of your own opinions and speculations. How can I show you Zen unless you first empty your cup?" (Reps & Senzaki, 1985, p. 19)

This story about an overflowing cup applies equally well to learning the principles and practices of DBT. The journey of learning is never easy, but traveling without extra baggage can help.

Like dialectics, Zen highlights the transient nature of reality, which ebbs and flows like waves in the ocean. In contrast to CBT procedures that teach clients how to actively change cognitions, affect, and behavior by using skills and other interventions, mindfulness and other practices drawn from Zen can help clients to observe how cognitions, affect, and impulses naturally develop and dissipate without any attempts to change them. These CBT and Zen approaches to problematic behaviors reciprocally enhance each other.

Zen practices focus on the current moment. Like CBT approaches, mindfulness teaches individuals to see reality without "delusions" (i.e., constructs, cognitive biases, or distortions) and to use skillful means. Zen practice emphasizes experience as the primary means of knowing the world. At some Zen monasteries, for example, novices learn the rules not from a printed list but from breaking them and experiencing the consequences. Consistent with dialectical principles, the practice encourages students to find a middle path.

DBT CONTEXT FOR BEHAVIORAL CHANGE

Diagnosis and Development of the Problem

Behavioral Approach to Diagnosis

DBT therapists maintain a behavioral conceptualization of diagnoses, considering a diagnosis of BPD or any other personality disorder as simply a label that summarizes a particular pattern of behaviors. If the behaviors cease, so too does the diagnosis. Furthermore, DBT therapists approach the diagnosis of BPD from a utilitarian perspective. DBT therapists do not "believe in" the diagnosis per se but use it because it has clinical utility. The empirical literature on BPD allows therapists to predict the prognosis of various types of treatments and to develop a treatment plan accordingly. Sharing the diagnosis with a client can communicate that the client is not "crazy" or "evil" or alone in having these problems and that change is possible.

Linehan reorganized the *Diagnostic and Statistical Manual of Mental Disorders, Fourth Edition* (DSM-IV; American Psychiatric Association, 1994) criteria for BPD into interrelated systems of dysregulation, namely affective, behavioral, cognitive, interpersonal, and self-dysregulation. The reorganized system applies equally to DSM-5 criteria

(American Psychiatric Association, 2013). Each system consists of conceptually related criteria, though the existence of one criterion does not necessarily increase the likelihood of another criterion within the same set (Heard & Linehan, 1994). Behavioral dysregulation includes suicidal and impulsive behaviors. Most DBT sessions, particularly early in treatment, focus on treating these types of behaviors. Affective dysregulation includes unstable emotions in general and anger in particular, while cognitive dysregulation consists of paranoid ideas and dissociation. Interpersonal dysregulation includes unstable relationships and problematic efforts to avoid abandonment, while self-dysregulation consists of an unstable sense of self and a persistent sense of emptiness.

Consistent with the emphasis in dialectics on the relationship among systems, DBT attends to how these systems of dysregulation influence one another and how interventions for one system can significantly change other systems. For example, emotional dysregulation in the form of frequent episodes of intense anger often destabilizes interpersonal relationships. Using new emotion regulation skills could lead to less anger *and* to more stable relationships. If someone has a relational sense of self, as many clients with BPD appear to have (Heard & Linehan, 1993), then instability in a relationship might destabilize the sense of self. Using new interpersonal effectiveness skills to solve interpersonal problems could stabilize interpersonal relationships *and* consequently the identity of the person with a relational self. DBT therapists particularly assess for any type of dysregulation that leads to a targeted behavior, and they then consider solutions for those types of dysregulation. For example, individuals who repeatedly engage in nonsuicidal self-injurious (NSSI) behavior most frequently identify affect regulation as its primary function (Klonsky, 2007; Nock & Prinstein, 2004). For unwarranted affect, both emotion regulation skills and exposure procedures can decrease the affect and consequently the related self-injurious behavior.

As described below in the biosocial theory, Linehan (1993a) hypothesizes that affective dysregulation plays a powerful, causal role in the problematic behaviors associated with BPD. Several studies have identified aspects of emotion dysregulation in BPD, including less emotional awareness and clarity (Leible & Snell, 2004; Levine, Marziali, & Hood, 1997), less willingness to tolerate distress in pursuit of a non-mood-dependent goal (Gratz, Rosenthal, Tull, Lejuez, & Gunderson, 2006), and greater use of emotional avoidance strategies (Bijttebier & Vertommen, 1999). Though research (Linehan, Tutek, Heard, & Armstrong, 1994) reveals that clients who are borderline tend to experience notably more anger than the population norm, experience also suggests that they have notable problems with other basic emotions as well (though client anger may prove the most problematic emotion for therapists). Thus, DBT therapists assess for problems with each of the basic emotions, rather than just for emotional dysregulation in general.

Linehan's conceptualization and treatment of affect depends on the work of emotion researchers (e.g., Gottman & Katz, 1990; Gross & Thompson, 2009). These researchers propose that emotional responses occur as a consequence of a prompting event or cue that an individual attends to and appraises as relevant to his or her goals. For example, if an individual attends to critical feedback from a boss or a loved one, interprets this feedback as disrespectful and has respect as a goal, anger will likely follow. If instead the individual ignores the feedback, interprets it as an attempt to help or does not care about the respect of the other person, then anger will not arise (assuming the absence of other appraisals or goals related to anger). An emotional response consists of a subjective experience, physiological changes, and behavioral components. The behavioral elements include cognitive behaviors, subtle facial expressions, body posture, and action urges, as well as more obvious overt behaviors. For example, an individual experiencing anger toward someone for acting disrespectfully may think judgmentally (e.g., "He shouldn't have said that," "He's stupid"), clench the jaw, stand rigidly, have urges to yell, and start an argument. Though a single emotion usually lasts only briefly, engaging in emotional behavior can prolong the experiencing of the emotion by repeatedly sending new emotional cues to the brain. Thus, continually thinking "He shouldn't have said that" repeatedly presents new anger-eliciting cues to the brain, long after the original critical feedback.

To treat problematic emotions, DBT therapists consider each contributing factor and element of the emotion as an opportunity for change. Therapists teach clients how to avoid or distract from unnecessary emotional cues, to challenge inaccurate appraisals or let go of ineffective ones, and to act opposite to the behavioral elements of an unwarranted emotional response. For example, if anger in response to critical feedback is unwarranted or ineffective, the individual could stop paying attention to the feedback, challenge the belief that the other person intends disrespect, let go of the goal of others always acting respectfully, mindfully let go of judgmental thoughts, think kind thoughts, do progressive relaxation for the face and body, or validate the other person instead of arguing. Furthermore, therapists balance helping clients to change ineffective emotions with teaching clients how to experience and tolerate potentially effective emotions.

Biosocial Theory

While classical and operant conditioning processes shape everyone's learned behaviors, Linehan (1993a) proposes that a developmental transaction between biologically based emotional vulnerability and persistently invalidating social environments provides the specific context in which these processes shape the behaviors that constitute the diagnostic criteria of BPD. This transaction results in clients' perpetual struggle to achieve emotional control. Linehan postulates that the criterion behaviors of BPD are either direct expressions of emotional vulnerability or the results of unskilled efforts to resolve the struggle. Linehan constructed DBT around principles and strategies to overcome the consequences of the continuing transaction between emotional vulnerability and invalidating environments.

EMOTIONAL VULNERABILITY

As part of the emotional vulnerability, Linehan highlights that individuals with BPD often experience a generally higher baseline level of emotional arousal. She also suggests that these individuals have a heightened sensitivity and reactivity to emotional cues, in which even relatively minor cues can evoke extreme responses. Finally, she proposes that a slow decay of emotional responses to baseline further compounds vulnerability to subsequent emotional cues. Jane, a woman in her early 20s, described these components of emotional vulnerability during her pretreatment interview (see Box 1.1).

INVALIDATING ENVIRONMENT

As part of the biosocial theory, Linehan (1993a) describes the characteristics and consequences of living in pervasively invalidating social environments, emphasizing their contribution to the development of behaviors associated with BPD. Using a "poorness-of-fit" model, she defines invalidating environments with respect to the environment's interactions with a particular individual rather than defining the environment independently from that relationship. Thus, an environment that consistently invalidates one individual may consistently validate another. Though individuals with BPD initially encounter invalidating environments during their childhood or adolescence, many also live in such environments as adults. Indeed, the mental health system can become another invalidating environment for many clients. Max, a young man presenting for treatment, described vividly all of the characteristics and many of the

---

Box 1.1. Jane's Emotional Vulnerability

During pretreatment, Jane's therapist inquired about her experience of emotion. Jane described her emotions as "intense" and "constant" and stated that she used self-harm to terminate the emotions and alcohol to "numb them out." She reported that the slightest thing can, and frequently does, "set me off" and that her responses to events are often "dramatic and over the top." Jane stated that family and friends confirm these self-descriptions. Indeed, she reported that her mother says that she responded in these ways as an infant, being more reactive to noise than any of her siblings and often startled by routine household sounds. Jane stated that she endeavors to manage her day and control her emotions by avoiding emotionally evocative or stressful situations and keeping social contact to a minimum. She added, however, that her efforts to manage in this way frequently fail and that even when they succeed they have a high cost: She has lost several jobs in recent years because of poor attendance because of her remaining at home to avoid emotional triggers. Jane described her emotional responses lasting a long time, even when triggered by relatively minor events (e.g., a sad story line in a television drama). The aftereffects of any emotional response seem, she reported, to make her vulnerable to further distress. She identified clearly that her pattern of harming herself regularly in the evening is often a desperate attempt to reregulate emotions so that she can sleep. Jane reported exhaustion with managing her emotions.

---

consequences of an invalidating environment in his own development (see Box 1.2).

Invalidating environments repeatedly communicate to the individual that his or her thoughts, emotions, urges to act, or actions, are essentially invalid ways of responding to the world. The environment also attributes these responses to socially undesirable personality traits. In effect, invalidating environments punish the individual for expressing internal experiences verbally or through other actions, consistent with Skinner's (1953) initial hypotheses of punishment as a mechanism of social control of behavior. The frequent punishment of such behaviors can then punish or at least extinguish related behaviors. Some individuals learn to ignore their own internal states because the environment's response does not reinforce such attention. Some individuals learn to punish their own internal experiencing by indiscriminately distrusting or judging these experiences. The environment's invalidation of internal responses also leaves individuals with notable skills deficits. For example, the capacity to understand affective responses derives from an

---

Box 1.2. Max's Invalidating Environment

Max described several ways in which his early upbringing failed to assist him to manage his emotional sensitivity. Max is one of four brothers, all of whom were much bigger and stronger than him. Each also excelled at sports, unlike Max. He described how his parents and his brothers frequently ridiculed him for being "weak and puny," and that when he cried or attempted to fight back the ridicule intensified. His elder brother, with his parents looking on and "approving" him being taught a lesson, frequently physically attacked him. Max reported becoming increasingly anxious and afraid during late childhood and early adolescence when he experienced further bullying at school where his brothers once again incited others to attack him. He worked hard to conceal his emotions as any display of distress initiated further criticism and hostility. In early adolescence, Max began drinking and smoking cannabis to excess to manage his increasing social anxiety, and he also discovered that cutting himself released some of his distress. He described that it was only when drunk that he had the courage to retaliate when his brothers became verbally hostile toward him. He described an occasion when he threatened his brothers with a serrated knife that previously he had used to cut himself. On this first occasion they backed down but subsequently started referring to him, at school and in the wider family, as "the family psychopath." Max gradually learned that he could stop verbal and physical hostility by producing a knife, harming himself in front of family members, or swallowing pills with alcohol in front of his family. Only on these occasions did family members desist from attacking him. Indeed, they would even access help from local health services on his behalf.

---

acknowledgment by others that the affective response has occurred, a normative labeling of the emotion, and an accurate explanation of its cause. As a result of emotional invalidation from a young age, clients with BPD frequently report persistent difficulties in recognizing and describing emotions, finding their own responses to events perplexing. Furthermore, successfully modulating affect requires the environment to teach a variety of skills; punishment alone does not suffice.

According to Linehan (1993a), invalidating environments shape two contrasting extremes of affective responses and then intermittently reinforce escalations of emotional expression. Individuals in invalidating environments commonly first respond with emotional inhibition to control affective responses. When inhibition fails either to regulate the affect or to initiate the desired environmental response, the individual may then escalate to extreme emotional behavior, either as a natural expression of affect or in an endeavor to reregulate the affective response. Sometimes the environment will ignore or possibly punish this extreme expression, but other times it will finally intervene to help the individual and inadvertently reinforce the escalation of emotional expression. When paired with the punishment of lower-level affective responses, intermittent reinforcement of emotional escalations teaches clients to oscillate between emotional inhibition and emotional escalation.

Invalidating environments communicate that the solution to life's vicissitudes involves simply trying harder or having more willpower. Such environments provide no constructive assistance in solving affective or other psychological problems, nor do they support and encourage an individual to tolerate the often painful journey of overcoming difficulties that cannot be immediately or simply resolved. This oversimplification can actually punish attempts to solve problems by increasing the likelihood that the individual will experience frustration, negative self-judgments (e.g., "I must be stupid"), shame or actual failure because of unrealistic expectations, and lack of problem-solving or coping skills.

Treating Capability and Motivation Deficits

Resolving the legacy of clients' early learning requires that DBT address any capability deficits in managing their highly sensitive, reactive affective systems and any motivational deficits inhibiting the client from engaging in more skillful behavior or motivating the client to engage in problematic behavior. Capability deficits addressed by the treatment focus on developing capacities to experience emotions without escalating or avoiding them; reducing unwarranted or ineffective emotions; maintaining interpersonal relationships despite intense affect; and maintaining flexible, mindful thinking despite high emotional arousal. In addition, assisting clients to acquire, strengthen, and generalize these new behavioral repertoires requires attention to motivational deficits. Invalidating environments tend to teach volitional motivational solutions to problems; this can be brutally summarized as "where there's a will there's a way." Such injunctions do not provide sufficient information on how to solve problems that defy easy or obvious solutions, nor do they provide sufficient skills and support to tolerate a problem that remains unresolved. Consequently, clients raised in invalidating environments experience frequent urges to give up on behavioral change. Therefore, DBT attends to and actively treats motivational problems as they arise, using a comprehensive behavioral approach to improve motivation.

A behavioral approach to motivational deficits focuses on assessing factors that impede the execution of new, more skillful behaviors (i.e., behaviors that are low in the client's response repertoire) and factors that reinforce or maintain target behaviors. Unwarranted affects, problematic cognitions, and punishing contingencies all inhibit the execution of new behaviors and discourage clients from persisting with solutions that over time, with sufficient rehearsal and reinforcement, would successfully resolve their difficulties. For example, a client who is obese needed to change two behaviors: decrease overeating, a behavior high in her existing behavioral repertoire, and increase exercise, a behavior low in her behavioral repertoire. Problematic emotions (namely, anxiety and sadness) and cognitions (namely, "No one wants me" and "It's hopeless") prompted overeating. Reductions in these emotions and thoughts, as well as a sense of comfort and warmth, reinforced overeating. Distal punishers of overeating included health problems and the client's dislike of her current weight. Whenever the client exercised, she experienced physical discomfort (breathlessness, muscle pain, sweat running down her face) that caused her anxiety about her physical health. Also, some types of exercise required her to leave the house, but when she left, her anxiety increased and she worried that others judged her for her weight issues. All of these consequences punished exercise. Distal reinforcements for exercise included praise from her doctor, whom she saw only monthly, and weight loss, if she consistently exercised. In this case the balance of reinforcement and punishment explains why overeating remained higher in the behavioral response hierarchy than exercise. Changing the client's motivation to decrease one behavior and increase the other required attention to treating both the antecedents and the consequences of the behaviors to shift the balance in favor of increased exercise and decreased eating. Thus, DBT therapists assess for emotions, thought, and contingencies that interfere with clients' motivation and treat them with exposure, cognitive restructuring, and contingency management, respectively.

Treatment Functions and Modalities

To treat the skills and motivational deficits described in the biosocial theory, Linehan has identified five primary functions or tasks of a DBT program. These tasks consist of enhancing client capabilities, improving client motivation, generalizing client capabilities, structuring the environment, and enhancing therapists' skills and motivation. Each task is addressed by one or more modalities of delivery (e.g., individual psychotherapy, psychoeducational group, telephone coaching), though the specific modalities vary according to the program's population and setting. Consistent with a dialectical approach, the different modalities of treatment depend on one another for success and can even shape one another. For example, in standard DBT the success of group skills training depends partly on how well the individual therapist helps the client further strengthen and generalize the skills. Client TIB during a skills training group may determine the agenda of the next individual therapy session. Therapist TIB during individual therapy may determine the agenda of the next consultation team meeting.

Standard DBT programs employ psychoeducational skills training groups (Linehan, 1993b) as the primary modality for enhancing capabilities. DBT skills trainers teach four modules or sets of skills, namely mindfulness, emotion regulation, interpersonal effectiveness, and distress-tolerance skills. Though the skills group has the primary responsibility for skills acquisition, and the beginning of skills strengthening and generalization, the individual therapist has the responsibility to teach the basics of any skills not yet covered in the group but immediately needed by the client, and to continue strengthening and generalizing the skills taught in group (e.g., suggesting skills as solutions to problems, rehearsing the implementation of those skills, integrating multiple skills).

In addition to having a repertoire of skills, successful problem solving requires sufficient motivation to act skillfully and a relative absence of motivation to act otherwise. Standard DBT primarily addresses the task of improving motivation in individual psychotherapy. The therapist and client complete behavioral chain analyses of targeted behaviors to determine the psychological and environmental factors motivating the client. They then implement cognitive restructuring, contingency management, exposure, and stimulus control procedures to decrease the factors that motivate the client's targeted behaviors and to increase the client's motivation to engage in skillful behavior. This book focuses primarily on problem solving within individual psychotherapy.

Consistent with behavioral approaches, DBT therapists do not assume that clients will automatically generalize newly acquired skills from therapeutic to real-life settings. The context of applying skills often differs substantially from the context of learning skills, particularly in terms of the client's degree of emotional dysregulation. DBT therapists emphasize the need for skills practice in all relevant contexts to generalize learning beyond the therapeutic context alone. Standard DBT programs offer clients the opportunity to telephone their respective individual therapists for brief skills coaching interventions between individual therapy sessions. These coaching calls focus on helping the client to apply skills to the current problem. Though clients can phone for skills coaching during a crisis, therapists encourage clients to phone before a problem becomes a crisis. Accessing coaching before a crisis seems to increase the number of possible solutions that clients can implement and to decrease the likelihood of therapist availability reinforcing crisis behaviors. To decrease the possibility of therapist availability reinforcing suicidal behaviors specifically, most DBT programs withdraw access to skills coaching for 24 hours after a suicide attempt or NSSI behavior. Research on the use of DBT telephone consultation (Linehan & Heard, 1993) suggests that DBT therapists do not receive significantly more calls compared with treatment-as-usual (TAU) therapists. Furthermore, the number of calls made by clients in the TAU condition correlated significantly with the combined number of their suicide attempts and NSSI, whereas no relationship between calls and these behaviors appeared in the DBT condition. Though the significant correlation could result from more suicidal clients phoning their TAU therapists more frequently, it may also be that TAU therapists increased their availability when clients phoned during suicidal crises or after suicide attempts or NSSI, thus potentially, though inadvertently, reinforcing these behaviors.

Structuring the environment focuses on helping clients to structure their natural environments in ways that prompt and reinforce the use of skillful problem solving and minimize aversive stimuli and the reinforcement of problematic behavior. The modalities used to address this function vary widely, depending on the program setting, the client population, and the individual client's particular environment. For example, inpatient programs may shape the milieu to address this function, whereas outpatient adolescent programs often involve the family. For a few adult outpatient clients, therapy sessions with a spouse may help to structure a more effective environment.

Finally, Linehan (1993a) strongly emphasizes the need for DBT programs to attend to the capabilities and motivation of DBT therapists. Treating the therapist as well as the client reflects the treatment's dialectical principles by attending to the two most important subsystems within the therapeutic context. Just as the therapist shapes the client's behavior, the client can shape the therapist's behavior. Unfortunately, many clients diagnosed with BPD intentionally or unintentionally shape therapists' behaviors in a detrimental direction, punishing therapeutic behavior or rewarding iatrogenic behavior. For example, a client might respond repeatedly with "I don't know" when the therapist attempts to conduct a chain analysis that elicits painful emotions, but then might speak freely if the therapist allows the conversation to distract to a less painful topic of the client's choosing. A client may express anger suddenly when the therapist suggests practicing a new skill but then may collaborate again if the therapist abandons skills rehearsal. In standard DBT programs, therapists employ weekly consultation team meetings to address the impact of clients' behaviors on therapists, as well as any other therapist motivational issues or capability deficits. Teams address a range of problems, including reviewing client target hierarchies, chain analyses and solution analyses, rehearsing the implementation of CBT procedures (e.g., cognitive restructuring, exposure), analyzing a therapist's urge to stop seeing a client, treating a therapist's TIBs (e.g., not balancing problem solving with validation, not implementing solutions in a session), and treating a therapist's consultation-interfering behaviors (e.g., missing consultation meetings, not participating during meetings). To treat these problems, the team applies the full range of problem-solving and other treatment strategies to each therapist.

Validation Strategies to Balance Problem Solving

Research has repeatedly reported that the efficacy of standard CBT treatments for various disorders declines significantly for clients with comorbid personality disorders. Compared with most clients who successfully complete a course of CBT, these clients have poorer treatment compliance and lower treatment retention rates. Linehan has suggested that the greater frequency of TIBs among clients with BPD occurs partially as a result of traditional CBT's strong emphasis on change, particularly in regard to changing one's own thoughts, emotions, impulses, and overt behaviors. She suggested that clients perceived the focus on change as not only invalidating of a specific response but as invalidating of their whole selves. Research by Swann, Stein-Serussi, and Giesler (1992) may explain how such perceived invalidation leads to TIB. Their research revealed that when someone challenges an individual's basic self-constructs, the individual's arousal increases. The increased arousal then leads to cognitive dysregulation and the failure to process new information. According to the biosocial theory, one would expect clients with BPD to have a heightened sensitivity to any potentially invalidating cues and a greater likelihood of becoming highly aroused in response.

Validation strategies serve as the main counterpoint to the change focus of problem solving within the treatment. DBT therapists validate clients' emotions, thoughts, urges, and actions that, crucially, are valid. Distilling valid responses amid a sea of dysfunctional behavior is a fundamental component of the treatment and provides the client with a different set of environmental responses to those experienced in past and current invalidating environments. Behaviors may prove valid or invalid in terms of their antecedents or their consequences (Linehan, 1997). For example, a client had an argument with her partner who threatened to leave her. She believed that he would leave, experienced extreme anxiety, and then cut herself, an action that decreased her anxiety and the attendant bodily tension. Upon discovering the cuts, her partner attended to her wounds. In this context, the anxiety certainly had validity as a consequence of the boyfriend's threat and her belief that he would leave; anxiety was a normative response to the antecedents. If the boyfriend did not plan to leave, the anxiety still would be a valid response to the invalid belief about the boyfriend leaving. The cutting had validity in terms of its short-term consequences in that it achieved the client's immediate goal of reducing anxiety and bodily tension, and it stopped the partner's threats of leaving. The cutting was invalid, however, in terms of the client's longer-term goals of learning to tolerate her emotions and of maintaining her relationship with her partner, who increasingly planned to leave her because of the cutting.

DBT therapists must disentangle the valid and invalid aspects of behavior in terms of the antecedents and consequences and clearly communicate these aspects to their clients. Linehan (1993a, 1997) describes two main types of validation, functional and verbal, that therapists use for this task. Many components of verbal validation consist of strategies familiar to therapists from a multitude of different therapeutic models. At its most basic, validation includes staying awake, literally and metaphorically, and observing even clients' most subtle verbal and nonverbal behaviors. Building on these observations, therapists validate by accurately describing what they observe to their clients. To treat clients' difficulties in understanding their internal experiences, therapists "read the patient's mind" (Linehan, 1993a), in the colloquial sense, by articulating clients' unverbalized thoughts, affects, sensations, and urges. As in many other therapies, DBT therapists may validate clients' behaviors in terms of the client's past learning or biological dysfunction. For example, when a client entered therapy with a history of multiple failed therapies, he expressed hopelessness about the prospect of DBT helping him. The therapist validated this by saying, "It makes sense you would be hopeless, as all other therapies that you've tried have failed." Validating in terms of biological dysfunction may relate to the biosocial theory or to ideographic biological issues for a particular client. For example, a client reported that she had experienced intense anger toward a family member over what she knew was a relatively minor issue. The therapist said, "That makes sense, as we know that people with BPD tend to have very sensitive emotional systems that lead to rapid and intense emotional reactions." A more personal historical validation with this client, who also happened to have poorly controlled diabetes, might be, "That makes sense because you always feel more irritable about things when your blood sugar is poorly controlled."

More distinctive of DBT are therapist communications that validate the client's behavior in terms of normative functioning or the current context and reflect "radical genuineness." Validating the client's behaviors in terms of the present context involves communicating to the client that his or her behavior makes sense because it is normal, reasonable, or effective in the current context. Thus, for the client discussed above with repeated previous unsuccessful therapies, a present context validation would be "I understand why you would worry that this therapy won't work, as this therapy is not effective for everyone, and we don't know yet if it is the most appropriate treatment for you." Frequently, clients experience present context validation as intrinsically more validating because of its nonpathologizing approach to their responses and histories. Dialectically, of course, both the present and past comments about the client's concerns about therapy have validity.

Radical genuineness requires DBT therapists to respond to clients as they would to any other person in their life who said, thought, or did what the clients said, thought, or did. In other words, therapists do not treat clients as highly fragile or volatile mental patients, but simply as individuals capable of learning to cope with therapists' responses. For example, when an adolescent client shamefully reported to her therapist that she had forced her younger sister to take amphetamines, saying she knew the behavior was wrong, the therapist said, "Makes sense to me you're ashamed. This is a major problem. What on earth were you thinking to do such a thing?" Therapists often find radical genuineness challenging as they have spent many years concealing their honest responses to clients' thoughts, emotions, and behaviors. DBT encourages therapists to strip away this concealment in the service of helping clients to improve their understanding of their own behavioral response and their impact on others. Radical genuineness validates the inherent capabilities of the client to learn to cope like nonclients with reality.

Therapists functionally validate when they act to help clients solve problems rather than just telling clients that they apprehend the seriousness of the problem. In this sense functional validation provides a direct route back to the problem-solving component of the treatment.

For example, a client who arrived disheveled at his therapy appointment reported that he had not had any suicidal urges during the week but had become homeless 2 days before. The therapist immediately said, "Okay, tell me what solutions have you tried so far. We have to solve this problem before you leave, and I don't want to waste time going over old ground." She then spent the session helping the client resolve his homelessness. Though the therapist's first comment did not concern the enormity of the problem or the client's emotional response, her immediate, unrelenting focus on solving the problem communicated to the client that she understood his dire circumstances.

Validation performs several functions in the treatment. Primarily, as indicated above, validation functions to balance the treatment's strong emphasis on change, which Linehan (1993a) identifies as particularly hard for clients with BPD to endure. In this sense validation sweetens the bitter pill of problem solving, the key ingredient of behavioral change in DBT. In addition to this main function, validation also provides feedback to the client about his or her behavior. This aspect of validation provides a useful counterpoint to clients' learning in invalidating environments that are characterized by the absence of accurate, nonjudgmental feedback about clients' behaviors and the behaviors' relationships to antecedents and consequences. Thus, validation provides clients with an opportunity for understanding their emotions, cognitions, sensations, and overt behaviors in their environmental context. Therapists also utilize validation to reinforce clinical progress. Research (Swann et al., 1992) has shown that humans significantly value validation and will work to achieve it. Thus, validating clients for collaborating in treatment, generating solutions, trying skills, or demonstrating progress will likely reinforce those behaviors. Finally, when validating clients, therapists model a key new behavior that they want clients to learn: self-validation. To persist in the long-term change process of therapy, clients require the capacity to validate their efforts to change, the emotional responses these efforts elicit, and the frustration that not having solved all their problems yet provokes. DBT therapists begin by modeling validation and then instruct clients to rehearse this skill for themselves. Dialectically then, even the core acceptance strategy has elements of change embedded within it.

CHAPTER 2

TARGETING

Selecting and Defining Problem Behaviors

CONCEPTUALIZATION AND STRATEGIES

During the initial case conceptualization in DBT's pretreatment stage, the individual therapist and client agree on which types of problems they will try to solve during treatment. DBT therapists then construct an individualized target hierarchy for their clients by translating clients' presenting problems and goals into behavioral targets and placing the targets at the correct point in the DBT treatment hierarchy. During subsequent sessions, the therapist helps the client to change the frequency of a problematic behavior (e.g., assaulting others, bingeing, cutting, dissociating, ridiculing other patients, starving, taking heroin) by focusing on or targeting a single episode of that behavior.

In contrast to many therapeutic approaches that allow clients to focus on whatever topic seems most important to them at the time of the session, DBT therapists select a specific target for analysis from a previously agreed-upon target hierarchy. Though some clients may experience this structure as invalidating, the structure serves several therapeutic purposes and the invalidation can be minimized by continually linking treatment targets to client goals and by shaping commitments to targets before placing them in the target hierarchy. By adhering to an agreed hierarchy, the therapist decreases the likelihood that the client's current mood or emotions determines the session agenda, thus decreasing the likelihood of reinforcing mood-dependent behavior. A hierarchy can also decrease the likelihood of therapists becoming overwhelmed by the number and changing nature of presenting problems. By including impulses or urges, as well as overt actions, in the target hierarchy, the treatment increases the likelihood of successfully treating a presenting problem rather than just suppressing it. Targeting a single episode enables the therapist to conduct a clearer BCA and better-matched solution analysis, resulting in a more accurate behavioral conceptualization. We begin by highlighting the key principles in constructing a target hierarchy during pretreatment and describe the procedures to select and define a target during a session. We then review common problems encountered in applying the principles of targeting and describe some potential solutions.

Construction of the Hierarchy in Pretreatment

Behaviorally Define Presenting Problems

Translating presenting problems into targets requires the therapist to define the problems behaviorally, that is, to describe the client's actual behavior in terms of what an observer would see or hear. Correctly defined behaviors give a clear picture to a stranger of precisely what the client does or says. A therapist may use a behavior's intent or consequences to categorize the behavior in the hierarchy or refine the definition but not as the definition. For example, NSSI is a category defined by the intent to physically harm oneself without dying, but the targets are cutting, burning, head banging, and similar behaviors. If a client phoned a therapist for skills coaching so frequently that it pushed the therapist's personal limits, then "phoning the therapist x times" would become the target because of the therapy-interfering consequence; the target would not be "pushes the therapist's limits."

Distinguishing behaviors from their motive or function is essential to effectively translating presenting problems into targets. Behavioral definitions preclude value judgments about the behavior or assumptions, or interpretations about the motive or function. For example, referrals for clients diagnosed with BPD sometimes describe the clients as "manipulative." Manipulative suggests a function for the behavior rather than providing a description of the behavior. Is the client threatening suicide if the therapist doesn't extend the session, telling conflicting narratives of events to the therapist and case manager, or making pottery skillfully? In addition to lacking clarity, confusing a description of the behavior with its function or motive increases the likelihood of conflict between the client and therapist. Based on fact, behavioral descriptions offer little opportunity for error or disagreement, but statements about motive, often based on interpretations, can easily prove erroneous or elicit disagreement.

Order Problem Behaviors in a Hierarchy

After therapists have defined a behavior, they must determine whether and where to place it on the DBT target hierarchy. Several principles help with this task: (1) categorize behaviors according to the hierarchy in the client's current stage of treatment, (2) include urges as well as actions, (3) include only behaviors that warrant the current stage of treatment, and (4) prioritize behaviors within categories. In the first stage of DBT, the relevant target hierarchy is the following:

1. Decrease suicidal behavior (e.g., suicide attempts, NSSI, suicide threats or planning, high urges to engage in these behaviors, significant increases in suicide ideation), homicidal behavior (e.g., murder or attempted murder, rape, physically attacking another with intent or consequence of serious harm, high urges to engage in these behaviors), and other imminently life-threatening behaviors (e.g., drinking alcohol when it could cause immediate kidney failure).

2. Decrease TIBs of both patient (e.g., missing sessions, leaving sessions early, not completing homework or implementing solutions, phoning beyond therapists limits) and therapist (e.g., failing to select a target for a session, not doing a chain or solution analysis, invalidating the valid).

3. Decrease severe "quality-of-life-interfering" behaviors, including psychiatric disorders "or other seriously destabilizing behaviors" (Linehan, 1993a); behaviors requiring intervention (e.g., arguing with spouse so loudly that neighbors call the police); or behaviors that significantly reduce global functioning scores (e.g., staying in bed all day).

4. Increase behavioral skills such as distress tolerance, emotion regulation, interpersonal effectiveness, and mindfulness.

DBT prioritizes life-threatening behaviors for the obvious reason of their high risk to life and because Linehan (1993a) originally developed the treatment specifically for suicidal behaviors. Less obviously, the treatment includes self-injury without suicide intent or imminent risk to life among the top targets because these behaviors predict subsequent suicide. DBT then targets TIBs to ensure that the client (and therapist) remains in treatment and to maximize the efficiency of treating any other target. Next, DBT treats psychiatric diagnoses and problems of similar severity because the treatment aims to help the client to achieve the client's goals and "a life worth living" (Linehan, 1993a), not just to become nonsuicidal but miserable.

As highlighted earlier, the top categories include impulses as well as actions to ensure the treatment of the target behavior, not just its suppression. The environment (especially controlled environments like hospitals and prisons) can dramatically reduce a target behavior simply by removing opportunities for it to occur or by punishing it. Such interventions can effectively reduce the behavior itself, such that the interventions appear to have solved the problem, but often they have succeeded only in suppressing the behavior. In such cases, the urges and the problems causing them remain, and the behavior often returns, especially if the context changes. Therefore, DBT treats high urges as well.

Next, the target hierarchy only includes behaviors sufficiently severe to warrant the client's current stage of treatment. Principles for determining if the behavior has sufficient severity for Stage 1 of DBT include whether the behavior poses an immediate physical risk to anyone, stops or notably impedes therapy, occurs as part of a psychiatric disorder, or requires intervention by authorities. Applying these principles present few challenges for therapists with respect to life-threatening behaviors as any behavior in this category is, almost by definition, appropriate for the first stage of DBT. Greater problems arise for therapists with regard to "quality-of-life-interfering" behaviors, as the category label may mislead therapists into thinking about more general quality-of-life issues, such as relationship satisfaction or balancing work and domestic life. DBT targets only those behaviors in this category that form part of a psychiatric diagnosis (e.g., bingeing, purging, dissociating), seriously destabilize the client (e.g., not taking diabetic mediation as prescribed), and require intervention or significantly reduce functioning. Thus, in Stage 1, DBT would target impulsively leaving a job, but not "being unfulfilled" by a job. Quality-of-life-interfering targets would include overeating that causes physical problems requiring medical intervention, but not simply wanting to lose weight in a client without physical problems.

Adherence to the target hierarchy does not mean that the therapy ignores clients' other issues. These other issues may be treated as links in the chain to a primary target or discussed separately after addressing the primary target in the session. They may become targets themselves if the client moves to an advanced stage of the treatment. For example, many clients in DBT report "low self-esteem" as a problem, but many people have low self-esteem and function well enough without any treatment. Despite not including self-esteem in the target hierarchy, the therapist would treat any related thoughts (e.g., "I'm worthless," "I'm useless") and emotions (e.g., shame) that appeared as causal links leading to targets in the hierarchy. Directly targeting low self-esteem would occur at a later stage of treatment, if needed.

Boxes 2.1 and 2.2 illustrate the transition from generic presenting problems to a DBT target hierarchy. Box 2.1 shows a referral letter for Jane, the client first introduced in Chapter 1. The letter contains some clear descriptions of behaviors (e.g., overdoses, binges, vomits, argues), some vaguely defined behaviors (e.g., self-harm, erratic attendance, argumentative), and some undefined problems (suicidal, chaotic relationships, unemployed). During pretreatment, the therapist further assessed and more behaviorally defined Jane's presenting problems and categorized the behaviors according to the target hierarchy as shown in Box 2.2. (For brevity, the box does not include Jane's many skills to increase.)

Box 2.1. Referral Letter for Jane

Re: JANE SMITH

Dear Dr. Hales,

I would like to refer Jane to your DBT program. Jane presents a number of management problems to our community team that we think your program could help to treat. She is diagnosed with borderline personality disorder and eating disorder not otherwise specified. She is frequently suicidal, having taken three overdoses in the last year, one of which resulted in admission to the intensive care unit. She also harms herself on a regular basis. Jane has binged and vomited on and off for the past 10 years. This pattern alternates with brief periods of eating restriction of anorectic proportions. Twice in the last 5 years with my team, her body mass index has decreased to below 17. Jane has chaotic interpersonal relationships, often arguing with family, friends, and mental health professionals. She is currently unemployed, having not worked for 3 years. It is my impression that it was her erratic attendance record and argumentative style that led to the termination of her most recent employment. She has attempted several types of psychological therapy over the years, none of which have helped her significantly. Despite these problems, Jane is a personable young woman who frequently asks for help with her many and varied problems.

Yours, etc.

Box 2.2. Jane's DBT Target Hierarchy

Life-Threatening Behaviors
  Suicide attempts:
  Overdosing

Nonsuicidal self-injury:
  Cutting of forearms, upper thighs, and stomach
  Vomiting to cause bleeding
  Burning forearms

Urges of four or more to engage in the above

Significant changes in suicidal ideation

Therapy-Interfering Behaviors
  Missing therapy appointments
  Refusing to practice suggested skills/problem solutions
  Threatening to tell therapist's manager and colleagues that therapist is
    incompetent
  Not concentrating in therapy sessions

Quality-of-Life-Interfering Behaviors
  Eating disorder not otherwise specified:
    Vomiting
    Bingeing
    Restricting food to fewer than 1,200 calories a day for more than a day

  BPD: Chaotic interpersonal relationships
    Threatening to disclose family's and friends' personal information that
      would cause them distress or embarrassment
    Threatening to report health professionals for incompetence when she
      dislikes their response

  Employment-related behaviors:
    Not applying for work currently
    Threatening boss and coworkers
    Missing many days at work

The referrer's description of Jane's interpersonal behavior particularly challenged Jane's therapist. The referrer described Jane as someone with an "argumentative style" and "chaotic" relationships. Neither of these problems has sufficient behavioral specificity, with the latter being a consequence rather than a behavior. Also, many individuals have slightly chaotic relationships or tend to argue, but these behaviors do not sufficiently destabilize their lives to warrant targeting at this stage of DBT. On inquiry the therapist discovered that many of Jane's arguments with family and friends constituted minor disagreements that did not destabilize the relationship. On some occasions, however, Jane threatened family and friends with publicizing personal matters that would embarrass or distress that person. This behavior resulted in frequent major disruptions with family members and friends and twice led to homelessness, albeit temporarily. Therefore, Jane's therapist targeted the threatening. Similarly with mental health professionals, Jane would threaten to inform their manager or colleagues that they were incompetent if she disliked their behavior. Jane's therapist anticipated that this may occur in their therapy relationship as well. They agreed to place threatening to complain about the therapist on the target hierarchy under "therapy-interfering behaviors."

To manage multiple targets within a category of the hierarchy, therapists and clients often develop a subhierarchy of target priorities. Therapists focus first on behaviors with the most severe, immediate consequences. Among the quality-of-life-interfering behaviors, Jane's therapist prioritized any episode of threatening that could leave Jane homeless and episodes of vomiting, which were causing longer-term physical damage. Consistent with CBT's emphasis on delivering evidence-based treatment, DBT therapists attend to targets that have empirically established efficacious treatments and emphasize these targets. Jane's therapist prioritized bingeing over restricting food partly because of a stronger evidence base for treating bingeing with DBT (e.g., Safer, Robinson, & Jo, 2010; Safer, Telch, & Agras, 2001; Telch, Agras, & Linehan, 2001). The client's motivation to address a target is certainly a critical factor. This was another reason for targeting bingeing before restricted eating in Jane's case. Similarly, the therapist and client may decide to prioritize easier problems to increase the likelihood of reinforcing therapeutic work. For example, one therapist and client decided to treat obsessive–compulsive behaviors before PTSD, as the therapist predicted an easier and faster course of treatment for the former and hoped that success in using exposure for the former would facilitate using it to treat the latter. Finally, therapists and clients may prioritize behaviors related to higher-order targets or the client's life goals. For example, one client had both substance abuse and clinically severe binge eating as quality-of-life-interfering targets, but only the bingeing increased her vulnerability to overdosing, so the treatment targeted bingeing before abusing substances. Because restricted eating frequently made Jane more vulnerable to suicidal behavior and bingeing, the treatment prioritized this target just after bingeing.

To assist the selection of the top target for each session and to track progress throughout treatment, clients record on a diary card each day their engagement in target behaviors. Though clients and therapists often collaboratively develop a personalized diary, all diary cards should include clients' top targets at a minimum. TIBs that the therapist can directly observe may not be recorded on the diary card unless recording them is part of the solution analysis. Initial diary cards may also track behaviors lower in the target hierarchy if those behaviors are a controlling variable for a higher target or the therapist has concerns that addressing a higher target will increase a lower target. As the therapy progresses to treating the lower targets directly, those targets are added to the card. Personalized diary cards often track variables, such as emotions, that contribute to target behaviors. Standard diary cards (Linehan, 1993a) also track skills use. Figure 2.1 shows the front of a diary card from early in therapy with Jane. The card has columns for Jane's top target of suicidal behaviors. The card generally does not record TIBs because these behaviors occurred in the therapist's presence, though Jane did use the verbal threat column to record any verbal threats to the therapist, as well as to anyone else. The card also has columns for the eating disorder behaviors. Not only were these the top quality-of-life-interfering behaviors (except for threatening that risked homelessness) and food restriction a vulnerability for suicidal behavior, Jane's therapist was concerned that Jane might suppress suicidal behaviors by increasing eating disorder behaviors.

Target Selection and Definition in Sessions

Select Target for Session According to the Hierarchy

The target hierarchy focuses the agenda of each individual therapy session, as well as describing the overall trajectory of treatment. Based on the client's target hierarchy and the behaviors reported by the client on the diary card for the past week, the therapist selects a single episode of the highest target as the priority for the session agenda. Traditionally, DBT requires clients to complete a diary card daily to monitor and report their top target behaviors and skills utilized during the week. At the start of the session, the therapist reviews the diary card, identifies the highest target that occurred during the preceding week and selects a specific incident or episode of that target behavior. Thus, the therapist would prioritize any incidents of suicidal or NSSI ahead of a therapy- or quality-of-life-interfering behavior.

Though therapists use a behavior's position in the target hierarchy

Diary Card — Jane — Completed in session? Yes/No — Date started: Monday, June 1

Day	Prescribed medication	Alcohol	Alcohol Specify	Suicide attempt or NSSI Urge (0–5)	Suicide attempt or NSSI Action: Y/N	Suicidal ideation 0–5	Verbal threats Urge (0–5)	Verbal threats Action: Who?	Vomiting Urge (0–5)	Vomiting Action: Y/N	Binges Urge (0–5)	Binges Action: Y/N	Restricting food Urge (0–5)	Restricting food Action: Y/N	Skills use 0–7
Mon.	As prescribed	0		2	N	1	0	N	2	N	3	N	3	N	5
Tues.	"	0		2	N	1	0	N	2	N	3	N	4	Y	4
Wed.	"	1	Vodka	4	Y—cut	3	5	Doctor	5	Y	4	Y	1	N	1
Thur.	"	0		2	N	2	0	N	2	N	2	N	3	N	5
Fri.	"	2	Beers	2	N	2	0	N	2	N	3	N	1	N	5
Sat.	8 NSAID	3	Glasses of wine	4	Y	5	4	Mom	3	N	4	N	1	N	1
Sun.	"	2	Beers	3	N	3	0	N	3	N	3	N	1	N	5

Skills Use:
0 = Not thought about or used
1 = Thought about, not used, didn't want to
3 = Thought about, not used, wanted to
4 = Tried but couldn't use them
5 = Tried, could do them, but they didn't help
6 = Tried, could use them, helped
7 = Didn't try, used them, didn't help
8 = Didn't try, used them, helped

Rating Scale for Emotions and Urges:
0 = Not at all; 1 = A bit; 2 = Somewhat;
3 = Rather strong; 4 = Very strong;
5 = Extremely strong

Urge to quit therapy before session: ___

FIGURE 2.1. The front of Jane's diary card.

as the primary determinant for selecting a target, this principle alone will not suffice if a client has multiple episodes of the highest target behavior (e.g., cutting on 3 days) or has episodes of different behaviors at the same point on the hierarchy (e.g., bingeing and smoking marijuana). In such instances the therapist and client would also consider the relative severity of the different episodes and the client's ability to remember and motivation to problem solve the different episodes. If the analysis of the top target does not require the full session, the therapy can then progress to another target or to other items on the client's agenda.

Jane's diary card reveals that several target behaviors occurred during the week. Jane cut on Wednesday and overdosed on Saturday. She also had one episode each of bingeing, vomiting, threatening to reveal something about her mother, and threatening her psychiatrist with filing a complaint. Based on Jane's target hierarchy, the therapist prioritized the overdose. After finishing the analysis of the overdose, the therapy then focused briefly on Jane's own agenda item of repairing her relationship with her psychiatrist. If no suicide attempt, NSSI, or related high urges had occurred during the week, the therapy would have assessed the relative severity of threatening the mother versus vomiting and then collaborated with Jane in selecting which of these behaviors to target.

Further Define the Session's Selected Target

Once the therapist and client have selected a specific episode of the target behavior to analyze, the therapist must then establish the precise form of the behavior during this episode. Although all targets in the hierarchy should have some behavioral definition, the therapist increases behavioral specificity at this point with respect to the form, severity, intensity, duration, and frequency. For example, if the client had cut, the therapist might assess the number of cuts, the length and depth of cuts, the amount and duration of bleeding, and what type of medical intervention had occurred. An assessment of bingeing might include details of the type and quantity of the food, the speed of eating, and the duration of eating. As in constructing the target hierarchy the therapist needs to describe the particular incident of the target behavior without inference regarding function. Examples of more specific behavioral descriptors include:

1. Life-threatening behaviors: Tied nylon cord around neck, attached the cord to hook on the back of the door, and had lifted her feet off of the floor before staff intervened. Cut a staff

member's forearm with a serrated plastic knife, making a cut approximately five inches long and half an inch deep.
2. TIB: Repeating "I can't do this" throughout a chain analysis.
3. Quality-of-life-interfering behavior: Hit partner across the face with her open palm, leaving finger marks on the partner's cheek. Vomited three times into the toilet in the bathroom; on the last occasion placed her fingers in her mouth and vomited mainly fluid that had specks of blood in it.

Such behavioral specificity serves several purposes. First, it helps to anchor the session in the target, consequently decreasing the likelihood that the session will drift away from the target. The specificity also decreases the likelihood that the session wastes time on a problem not in the hierarchy. Finally, such an assessment can help to determine which episode to select when multiple episodes of a single behavior type appear on the diary card.

COMMON PROBLEMS

Correctly employed, targeting simplifies the task for the therapist in deciding the session agenda and facilitates the effective commencement and continuation of the BCA. If the therapist fails to properly select and define a target behavior at the beginning of the session, however, the chances of successfully conducting a chain and solution analysis decrease dramatically. Several TIBs interfere with targeting fulfilling its function. These TIBs may arise as a result of conceptual confusion about the principles of targeting or how to apply them. These TIBs can include a lack of mindfulness or motivation in applying targeting strategies or problematic emotions that derail the therapy, despite a comprehensive understanding of targeting. Problems with target selection are reviewed next followed by problems with target management.

Not Reviewing the Diary Card

Not requesting a diary card or not receiving one upon request obviously impedes the selection of the top target for the session. If a client did not bring a completed diary card, the first and most simple solution is to present the client with a blank diary card and request that he or she complete it. This response often provides a good opportunity for therapists to assess problems with diary completion as they occur and a useful contingency for clients who otherwise find not completing the card reinforcing. In many instances, the client completes the diary card and the session proceeds as usual, though the therapist might inquire briefly about the problems leading to the initial absence of the diary card and troubleshoot with the client how to prevent the problems from reoccurring. If the client repeatedly fails to bring a completed diary card, the therapist would include the behavior on the target hierarchy as an out-of-session TIB and treat the behavior accordingly. For example, if an analysis indicated that the client repeatedly forgot to complete the diary card during the week, the therapist would help the client to develop cueing strategies, such as scheduling a regular time each day to complete the card or creating environmental cues (e.g., Post-it Notes or cell-phone reminders).

If a client refuses to complete the diary card on request, the therapist then uses problem-solving strategies to treat this behavior. By using a brief BCA, the therapist assesses the clients' emotions, thoughts, and behaviors related to completing the diary card. Common controlling variables include not remembering behaviors across the week and overwhelming affect that inhibits thinking, writing, or talking about the week. With regard to overcoming the memory problem sufficiently for that session, the therapist can work through the week by starting with the session day and moving backward or by focusing on the days that likely had more memorable events (e.g., attending group) or about which the therapist already knows something (e.g., due to a phone call). Typically, the further away from the session, the more difficulty the client experiences with recollection. In these circumstances, as soon as an episode of a higher-priority target behavior appears, the therapist can switch from completion of the diary card to analysis of the higher-priority behavior. Switching away for a lower-order target (e.g., increased depressed mood) runs the risk of failing to analyze a higher-order target that noncompletion of the diary card conceals.

Most often, affect interferes with diary card completion, in session and out of session alike. For example, early in therapy, Susan frequently did not complete her diary card at home and refused to complete it during sessions. On presenting the diary card to Susan for completion in session, her therapist observed that Susan looked away and said, "I can't do it! Everything is pointless." A mini-chain analysis of this sequence revealed that the request to complete the card elicited shame. Susan confirmed that shame also prevented her from completing the card during the week. When faced with the diary card in therapy and at home, Susan ruminated about her problematic sexual behavior, her own untrustworthiness, and her view of herself as a "hopeless case." Naturally, these cognitions fueled her shame, which she initially tried to avoid by not completing the diary card. In response, Susan's therapist treated the in-session refusal to complete the diary card by using exposure procedures (see Chapter 6). After completing the diary card, Susan and her therapist discussed how to generalize the exposure procedure to the completion of the diary card at home.

Not Selecting a Target or Using the Hierarchy for the Selection

As discussed earlier, the target hierarchy, diary card, and targeting strategies guide therapists in selecting a single episode of behavior for analysis. Sometimes, therapists fail to benefit from these elements of the treatment because they fail to select a target at all or to use the target hierarchy. A BCA might reveal that the TIB occurred because the therapist did not remember the various elements of targeting, the therapist dismissed the importance of or disagreed with the target hierarchy or targeting strategies, the therapist received insufficient reinforcement for treating a particular target, or emotions interfered with the application of the targeting strategies. The therapist or consultation team would then generate and implement solutions that correspond to the variables causing absence of targeting or applying the target hierarchy. For example, novice therapists who simply do not remember to select a target may benefit from working through a "How to start a session" checklist at the beginning of each session. A therapist who does not remember the target hierarchy may benefit from reviewing a copy of the client's hierarchy at the beginning of the session. If a therapist has treated a client's top target in a number of sessions, but the behavior has not changed, the therapist may experience insufficient reinforcement to persist with the target. In such a case, the team could increase the therapist's reinforcement by praising or validating the therapist for persisting in choosing the top target. They might also encourage the therapist to measure short-term success according to the therapist's adherence to the model rather than the client's outcomes. Of course, if the team helps the therapist to treat the top target more effectively, the therapist will certainly experience more reinforcement.

In one case a therapist failed to follow the target hierarchy because he disagreed with the treatment principles that underpin the hierarchy. More specifically, he disagreed about placing cutting near the top of the hierarchy as he considered it less serious than some of the client's quality-of-life-interfering behaviors. After the team noticed the therapist's TIB, they first tried reviewing the rationale for applying the hierarchy (i.e., this category of behavior remains the best predictor of subsequent suicide, changing the targeting priority deviates from the evidence base for the treatment). When this solution proved insufficient, the team helped the therapist to develop willingness and radical acceptance of the treatment as it is and to mindfully let go of urges to "rebel." They also applied some contingency management, which included expressing more interest in the therapist when he used the target hierarchy and cool confrontation when he failed to do so.

Emotions often lead therapists to abandon the established target hierarchy and thus interfere with targeting. Because of emotions such as shame, fear, or anger, clients sometimes become noncollaborative about selecting the highest target for analysis. In some instances, therapists can treat the refusal or similar behavior with minimal behavioral conceptualization and intervention. For example, simply linking the target to a client's long-term goals may sufficiently increase the client's willingness to tolerate moderate shame elicited by the targeting. At other times, treating the client's TIB may require a more comprehensive BCA and solution analysis. In either instance, clients can learn through the process of treating such behaviors. Unfortunately, a client will learn the wrong lesson if the therapist bases the selection of a target on his or her own emotional responses to the target itself or to the client's initial noncollaboration. Therapists' most common emotions that interfere with targeting seem to consist of fear, guilt, and interest. Any negative emotion, however, can cause therapists to avoid targeting certain behaviors, thus preventing clients from receiving treatment for those behaviors. By avoiding particular targets, clients and therapists alike are negatively reinforced by any reduction in their negative emotions, thus perpetuating avoidance as a therapeutic strategy. Resolving this pattern of avoidance requires that either the therapist or the consultation team notice and treat the behavior.

Max had a history of making allegations of bullying whenever therapists confronted him about certain behaviors. As a consequence, Max had "burnt out" several therapists. Although during pretreatment Max had agreed to address his self-harm behaviors, targeting this behavior became a challenge early in treatment. Whenever Max's therapist endeavored to target self-harm behaviors, Max became angry and started shouting at her, accusing her of incompetence. Frightened by Max's aggressive behavior and doubting her own competence, the therapist began to avoid targeting self-harm behaviors and did not confront Max about his TIBs. Members of her team noticed this problem and treated the therapist's avoidance with several strategies. Of particular note, the team reviewed the therapist's own behavioral chain of her avoidance and identified that thinking "Maybe this is too difficult for him, and it would be better to focus on less painful issues" and "Perhaps he's right that I'm not doing this well" interfered with her willingness to target self-harm. The team helped the therapist to increase her mindfulness of these thoughts, to challenge them with cognitive restructuring, and to refocus her attention on her goal to implement adherent DBT and Max's goal to overcome his increasingly dangerous and risky self-harm. Recognizing that she did not have a sufficient analysis of Max's aggressive outbursts, the therapist reviewed the sequence of events that occurred in therapy and generated some hypotheses about problematic links in the chain. She then role-played how to address the aggressive outbursts with Max. During their session, the therapist described to Max the pattern of their mutual TIBs; in other words, she behaviorally defined the problems. She described her concerns that failure to resolve the problem would prevent Max from reaching his goals (i.e., she linked the target to his goals and clarified the contingencies), while at the same time validating his urge to avoid. Using her earlier hypothesis generating as a guide, she and Max analyzed the factors leading to his aggressive outbursts and generated and rehearsed relevant solutions. Within two to three sessions, Max tolerated chain analyses of self-harm notably better, and directly told his therapist whenever he experienced urges to avoid any discussion.

Therapists can also deviate from the session agenda as a result of positive emotions such as happiness or interest. As with other TIBs, treating these behaviors requires an understanding of and implementing solutions for the variables controlling the behavior. Although this set of behaviors requires treating an emotion that therapists want to keep rather than avoid, therapists can still use the same solutions for the emotions. For example, one therapist with an extensive family therapy background tended to prioritize family-related problems over the target hierarchy. An analysis of this TIB revealed that the therapist experienced greater happiness discussing family issues, primarily because she experienced great confidence when she focused on this topic. The team helped her to become more mindful of her emotions and urges, to surf the urge, to let go of her attachment to experiencing confidence and happiness, and to radically accept not being confident at that moment.

Failing to Define the Problem Behaviorally

Either during the development of the target hierarchy or the selection of an episode of a target, therapists can fail to define the target with enough behavioral specificity. For example, "aggressive" does not provide a sufficient description for someone to imagine the client's specific actions, which could range from yelling to throwing furniture to hitting someone. When one therapist listed "decrease dependence" as a TIB, the consultation team highlighted that this phrase did not describe the form of any behavior. They then helped the therapist to describe specific behaviors that actually interfered with the therapy, such as "phoning the therapist every day," which stretched the therapist's limits. Claire's therapist described her adolescent client's behavior as "passive" in session, but she had difficulty treating this TIB. As a first step, the team suggested that she more clearly define the target behavior(s), so that the therapist and Claire knew precisely what behavior(s) needed to increase or decrease and had a clearer focus for their analyses. Claire's refined targets consisted of "automatically responding with 'I don't know,'" "not using skills during the week," and "asking therapist to solve environmental problems" for her.

Occasionally a therapist might erroneously target another person's behavior rather than the client's. For example, a therapist might inadvertently focus on a boyfriend abusing a client rather than the client returning to live with the abusive boyfriend or the client cheating on the boyfriend. The focus on the client's behavior does not blame the client for the abuse; it simply acknowledges the reality that therapists can only treat individuals who seek treatment.

More commonly, therapists mistakenly define the target by the consequences or function rather than the form of the behavior. Many presenting problems describe the consequences of a behavior or set of behaviors rather than the behavior itself. For example, "unemployed" describes someone's employment status, not the behaviors that caused the status. Possible target behaviors include refusing to apply for jobs, disclosing too much personal information during interviews, arguing with bosses, and impulsively quitting jobs. Similarly, "homeless" only describes someone's housing status. Possible targets might consist of not paying rent and violating public housing drug policy. "Marital discord" describes the state of a relationship not the interpersonal behaviors that caused that state. Specific targets might include assaulting the spouse, spending the family's limited money on expensive items for oneself, and arguing daily with the spouse. When one therapist listed "decrease alienating caregivers" as a target, the consultation team highlighted that this phrase described a consequence rather than a behavior. They then helped the therapist to identify the behaviors that led to this consequence, namely "yelling at caregivers" and "not answering the door to caregivers."

When therapists define a target by the consequences of a behavior, they often focus particularly on the functional consequences. For example, one therapist listed "decrease avoidance" as a TIB. The consultation team highlighted that this phrase described the function of a behavior, rather than an actual behavior. The therapist then identified "missing the skills training group" as the actual behavior. Therapists sometimes compound the error of confusing behaviors with their functions by assuming rather than assessing the function of the behavior. For example, the case manager who referred Claire to DBT stated that Claire had a tendency to "split" her clinicians and family. Claire's DBT therapist simply included this problem in the target hierarchy, but when she reviewed the hierarchy with the team, they immediately identified two problems. First, "split" does not describe the form of any behavior in a way that anyone else could imagine what Claire actually did. Second, the term derives from theoretical assumptions about the function of the behavior. With coaching from the team, Claire's therapist described the actual form of the problematic behavior. She identified that Claire had a pattern of describing personal events in radically different ways to different members of her clinical network and family. In one episode of the new target, Claire had cried profusely and reported high suicidal ideation to her psychiatrist only a day or two after reporting significant improvement to her case manager. An analysis of the actual reasons for these different responses revealed that the behavior did not function to split the clinicians, even if it had that consequence. Instead, Claire described "editing" accounts of distressing events depending on how she thought the other person would react. She particularly feared that her case manager would judge her for her more extreme behaviors, whereas her psychiatrist tended to respond with lots of validation and soothing.

Though any error in behavioral definition can reduce the effectiveness of the ensuing BCA, inferences about the intent or function of the behavior can also cause conflict in the therapy relationship. In one case, the staff on a standard inpatient unit described their patient Rita as "attention seeking." This label summarized their assumptions about the intent or function of Rita's actions on the unit, but it did not describe the behaviors themselves. Without identifying the actual behaviors, Rita's DBT therapist told Rita that they needed to target her "attention-seeking behavior." Rita immediately became angry and denied that she engaged in such behavior. The therapist described threatening to complain about staff, teasing other patients, and playing music loudly, using these examples as evidence of seeking attention. Rita admitted to the behaviors, but continued to deny seeking attention. The session had become rather

polarized when the therapist realized that she had confused the identification of a target behavior with assumptions about the function of
the behavior. After apologizing, the therapist refocused the session on
an episode of Rita's teasing another patient and discovered through the
behavioral analysis that the behavior actually reduced Rita's fear by
decreasing the likelihood that other patients would challenge her.

Selecting an Incorrect Target Due to a Conceptual Error

Even with a good behavioral definition, therapists can still target incorrectly if their target hierarchy contains conceptual errors. These errors
include failing to consider strong urges as targets, placing behaviors in
the wrong target category, and confusing links in the chain with the target itself. Such conceptual errors may prove difficult for the therapist to
detect, as they do not have an immediate negative impact during the session, despite their potential negative long-term impact. The consultation
team may have the best chance of detecting conceptual problems and
therapists should review at least new target hierarchies with the team.

A lack of clarity about which behaviors comprise which target category can lead therapists to place a behavior too high or too low in
the target hierarchy. For example, therapists may hesitate to prioritize
NSSI (e.g., scratching, head banging) in the top category, if they focus
on the overarching category label of "life-threatening," rather than the
subcategory of suicidal behavior, which includes all types of NSSI. Alternatively, therapists may assume that because a behavior causes some
form of harm that it automatically counts as a "self-harm" behavior
and ranks in the top category of life-threatening behaviors. For example, therapists occasionally place vomiting under the top target because
it causes bodily harm. Vomiting, however, is seldom imminently life-
threatening or suicidal, as individuals typically do not intend to cause
bodily harm. Instead, the harm is incidental to the primary aim of purging and weight loss. If the client intends self-harm through vomiting,
such as Jane who occasionally vomited in order to make her esophageal
lining bleed, then the vomiting would count as NSSI. In the case of the
client whose potassium level often fell dangerously below normal levels,
any vomiting could have caused an imminent risk to her life and thus
counted as a life-threatening target. As her physical state improved and
her potassium level returned to normal, vomiting returned to a lower-
level priority under quality-of-life-interfering behaviors.

Distinguishing a target behavior from a link in the chain to the
target behavior presents a challenge for many therapists. For example,

one therapist listed "discouraged about treatment" as one of the client's TIBs. The team suggested that discouragement need not inherently interfere with the treatment and suggested that it may be a link leading to a behavior that directly interfered with the treatment. The therapist then identified the actual TIB as canceling therapy sessions. Behavioral chain analyses of canceling revealed links related to discouragement, but it also revealed other important controlling variables for canceling. In another case, a therapist listed "fears abandonment" as a quality-of-life-interfering behavior. The team highlighted that fearing abandonment did not directly destabilize anyone's life, require intervention, or lead to a low functioning. They helped the therapist to identify the actual target behaviors as "calling husband repeatedly at work," which jeopardized his job and the couple's financial stability, and "crying profusely when husband wants to spend time without her," which severely destabilized their marriage.

In some cases, the incorrectly identified target might be a target further down the hierarchy, but is only a link to a higher-priority target. For example, under "therapy-interfering behaviors," a therapist might list "insomnia," "abusing drugs," or "anorectic behaviors," as any of these problems can impact a client's participation during sessions. DBT requires, however, that therapists precisely specify the behavior that directly impedes effective engagement in therapy. Examples of such behaviors include "falls asleep in session," "does not remember solutions generated after the session," and "does not process information during the session." A chain analysis of any of these targets might reveal poor sleep, drug misuse, or inadequate nutrition as relevant links in the chain, but the therapist would need to assess the extent to which they actually control the target behavior. Many people sleep poorly, for example, but manage to stay awake throughout meetings. Crucially, other links may have a stronger impact on the target or offer better opportunities for implementing solutions. By focusing on a single link rather than the sequence of links to the specified target behavior, therapists risk missing other relevant controlling variables and thus restricting the choice of viable solutions.

In one case, a client, whose hierarchy included cutting and abusing alcohol, began to arrive significantly late to therapy. The therapist correctly assumed that the client had started drinking before the session and thus decided to target the drinking, but neither the drinking nor the tardiness stopped. The consultation team highlighted the therapist's targeting error and refocused her analyses on the tardiness instead of the drinking. The chain analysis now revealed other key controlling variables, including that the client lost track of time before the session, partly due to the alcohol and partly due to general disorganization. In contrast to solutions for the drinking, environmental solutions that reminded her of the time (e.g., alarms, phone calls from others) notably decreased the tardiness. If no TIB had occurred, then the therapy progressed down the hierarchy to targeting an episode abusing alcohol. Thus in some cases, an identified link to a high target eventually becomes a lower-order target itself.

Distracting from or Not Returning to the Target

Adherent DBT sessions require good discipline throughout the session. Sometimes, therapists successfully begin a session by identifying and beginning to treat the correct target, but later lose the discipline by moving away from the target, never to return to it again. Quite correctly, the therapist may suspend the analysis of the selected target if the client has begun to engage in a TIB that requires immediate treatment. Unfortunately, therapists also change focus for less therapeutic reasons or in less therapeutic ways. Some therapists distract away from the original target when clients mention other crises in their lives or topics that particularly interest the therapist. Other therapists decide to abandon behavioral chain analyses when clients communicate that the analyses distress them or that they do not want to do the analyses. Moving away from the behavioral chain analyses in any of these circumstances, however, may inadvertently reinforce clients' TIBs. Unfortunately, it may also relieve therapists and consequently reinforce their nonadherent behaviors too! Preventing the distraction or avoidance requires therapists to remain mindful of the target and to treat their own emotions (e.g., fear, interest, guilt) and impulses (e.g., abandon the analysis), usually by acting opposite. Dysfunctional cognitions (e.g., "I must focus on today's housing crisis instead of yesterday's cutting," "This is too distressing") may also require treatment. Contingency management from the team usually helps to counteract any relief experienced by the therapist for avoiding or any punishment from the client for not avoiding. In some cases, a client's problematic in-session behavior will stop if the therapist simply continues with the analysis. More severe or persistent TIBs, however, often require direct treatment and a *temporary* suspension of work on the original target.

After treating in-session behavior, therapists sometimes fail to return to the original target. This problem occurs commonly when therapists "become lost" in the analysis and treatment of the in-session behavior and forget the original target or its links. In these circumstances, listening to therapy tapes can assist therapists in identifying when precisely the problem occurs. Solutions may involve keeping notes during the therapy session of the main chain and developing increased mindfulness of the therapy process. At other times therapists do not return to the original target because treating the in-session behaviors required so much effort or elicited so much affect that the therapists literally feel exhausted. Mindfulness in these circumstances can decrease the likelihood or impact of fatigue, and more practice can further increase endurance, just as it does with athletes. A literal or figurative "stretch break" can revive therapists and clients alike. Some therapists also worry that if they return to analyzing the original target, the TIB will return as well. From a DBT perspective, the therapist has little to lose from returning to analyze the original target and much to lose from not returning. Even if the return does elicit more TIBs, the therapy can then refine the solutions for those behaviors.

CHAPTER 3

BEHAVIORAL CHAIN ANALYSIS

CONCEPTUALIZATION AND STRATEGIES

DBT therapists use behavioral chain analyses (BCAs) to determine the function of a target behavior and to identify the causal relationships among the psychological, overt behavioral, and environmental events immediately preceding and following the behavior. After selecting a single episode of a target behavior, the therapist commences a BCA of the behavior. The therapist and client identify the links in the chain by assessing the sequence of affects, cognitions, impulses, actions, and environmental events that led to and resulted from that selected episode, with a particular emphasis on the links most proximate to the target. Critically, the therapist must also *analyze* this chain to evaluate the causal relationships among the links and to identify particularly those links that control the target behavior. Though the insight provided by such an analysis can prove directly beneficial, the BCA serves primarily to provide the prerequisite information for selecting links to treat in the solution analysis. This chapter reviews the structural, theoretical, and strategic aspects of a competent BCA and then discusses common problems in each of these areas. Solution analyses are discussed in Chapter 4.

Structure of a BCA

Structural principles help therapists to identify the beginning and end-points of the chain and to describe accurately the links in the episode. A behavioral chain is not simply a narrative of the client's day; instead, it analyzes a relatively brief time period determined by the escalation and resolution of the urge to engage in the target behavior. The cases in Boxes 3.1, 3.2, and 3.3 demonstrate this difference. For each case, the first box (3.1a, 3.2a, and 3.3a) provides a simple narrative involving a target behavior (overdosing, vomiting, and threatening to file a complaint, respectively). The second box for each case (3.1b, 3.2b, and 3.3b) articulates the BCA for the target. In comparing the two accounts, the narrative version places a greater emphasis on earlier events in the sequence, events that the BCA would identify as vulnerability factors. For example, the arguments with the boyfriend and the therapist, anxiety about the relationship with the boyfriend, and drinking mentioned in Box 3.1a are listed as vulnerabilities in Box 3.1b. In contrast, the BCA emphasizes the later psychological links that the narrative somewhat neglects. A complete chain can cover a brief period of only a few minutes, but most cover periods of at least 20 minutes. Analyses of periods of several hours may indicate that the BCA has become mired in a narrative or vulnerability factors. Focusing on the links close to the target behavior requires therapists to limit attention to other behaviors or events that either especially interest the client (the relationship with the boyfriend in Box 3.1) or the therapist (the therapeutic rupture in Box 3.1). To minimize the chances of eliciting a narrative or focusing too much on vulnerability factors, therapists generally start analyses with questions that focus on the target or its proximate links, such as "What was happening just before you cut?" and "When did you first notice

---

Box 3.1a. Susan's Narrative

At lunchtime, Susan argued with her boyfriend over the phone. He hung up and she began to worry that he would end the relationship. She reminded herself that she could discuss this with her therapist later in the afternoon. During the therapy appointment, the therapist agreed to add Susan's relationship to the agenda but would not prioritize it over the analysis of parasuicidal behavior that occurred earlier in the week. This angered Susan. Still anxious about the relationship with her boyfriend, Susan phoned him that evening to repair the relationship, but he didn't answer the phone. She then went out drinking with a friend. After a couple of drinks, she agreed to go home with a man who she had just met. They had sex and immediately after, Susan felt "bad" about cheating on her boyfriend. She then overdosed on her prescription medication. The man realized what happened, phoned the paramedics, and left. Susan received medical treatment at the hospital and was admitted to the psychiatric ward.

Box 3.1b. BCA of Susan's Overdose

Target: Takes 30 antidepressant pills.

Function of the target: Reduce guilt and shame and reestablish connection with the boyfriend.

Vulnerability factors	Argument with her boyfriend, thinks relationship will end and feels anxious.
	Disagreement with individual therapist and feels anger.
	Drinking.
	Agrees to take a male stranger home and feels happy.

Type of link	**Link in chain**
Prompting event	Has sex with man at home.
Cognition	Thinks, "I shouldn't have sex with someone else."
Affect	Guilt (4/5).
Impulse	Urge to self-harm (3/5).
Cognition	Thinks, "I'll feel better if I harm."
Action	Curls up in bed.
Environmental event	Hears man move.
Cognition	Thinks, "I'm a cheat."
Affect	Guilt increases (5/5), shame (5/5).
Cognition	Thinks, "I don't deserve him anyway."
Cognition	Thinks, "I don't even deserve to live."
Impulse	Urge to self-harm increases (4/5).
Action	Goes to the bathroom to overdose.
Target behavior	Takes 30 antidepressant pills.
Negative reinforcement	Guilt decreases (3/5), shame decreases (3/5).
Sensation	Nausea and wooziness.
Environmental event	Man enters bathroom, appraises situation, calls paramedics, and leaves.
Sensation	Nausea and wooziness continue.
Environmental event	Paramedics arrive, administer treatment, and take her to the hospital.
Environmental event	Is assessed and admitted to the psychiatric ward.
Cognition	Thinks, "I deserve being stuck here as a punishment."
Negative reinforcement	Guilt decreases (2/5).

(continued)

Box 3.1b. (*continued*)

Later consequences	
Environmental event	Boyfriend visits and tells her that he's learned the "whole story," but forgives her because she "must have been really sorry" if she "tried to kill" herself.
Negative reinforcement	Guilt decreases (1/5), shame decreases (2/5).
Positive reinforcement	Experiences strong connection to boyfriend.

the urge to overdose increase above its baseline?" Similarly, to maintain the focus on a single episode of the target therapists minimize questions that draw clients into summarizing what "usually" occurs. For example, Susan's therapist did not ask, "How do you feel after having sex with a stranger?" Instead, she focused on the specific targeted episode by asking, "What emotions and thoughts did you experience immediately after having sex with the man Tuesday night?"

Chain analyses begin with a prompting event and end with the consequences of the target behavior. Most prompting events involve a new or altered stimulus in the client's external environment, such as a parent criticizing the client's actions, a repossession notice arriving in the mail, or a fellow prisoner pushing into the lunch line. In some instances, however, internal stimuli, such as auditory hallucinations or nightmares, prompt a target behavior. Strategies to more accurately locate the prompting event include asking when the urges to engage in the target behavior first occurred and then assessing for the most proximate environmental event. It may also prove helpful to establish the event on which the subsequent chain depended, such that if the event had not occurred, then the target behavior would not have occurred. In the chain analysis displayed in Box 3.1b, Susan was sure that without the sex with a stranger she would not have overdosed; none of the other events, either alone or in combination, would have resulted in the overdose. These other events—namely, the argument with the boyfriend, the disagreement with the therapist, and her boyfriend not answering his phone—all constitute vulnerability factors. Though starting the chain analysis with an assessment of the prompting event is logical, therapists may decide to start the chain with another link and work backward to the prompting event. If these strategies produce no clear prompting event, the therapist should progress with the rest of the chain analysis, as successful problem solving requires enough links in the chain and enough time for the solution analysis, rather than a perfect chain analysis.

Therapists need to obtain information on both environmental *and* psychological consequences of the target behavior, especially with regard to affect regulation. A comprehensive chain analysis includes an assessment of both immediate and more distal consequences. In Susan's case, her overdose immediately resulted in decreased guilt and shame. Later, when her boyfriend forgives her, she experiences a further decrease in guilt and shame and a strong connection to her boyfriend. Because the assessment of the consequences provides one of the best opportunities for insight into the function of the target behavior, therapists who tend to miss assessing consequences may benefit from starting their chain analyses with at least a brief assessment of the immediate consequences.

A chain analysis also requires therapists to specify the psychological and environmental links between the prompting event and the immediate consequences of the target behavior. Therapists must disentangle the often overwhelming confusion of inner experience and environmental chaos into a series of smaller, specified, linear links, mindfully reviewing clients' experiences "frame by frame." Therapists differentiate environmental events, cognitions, affects, sensations, impulses, and overt actions from one another and then label these links, as Boxes 3.1b, 3.2b, and 3.3b illustrate. Whether done verbally or in writing, labeling the types of links enables therapists and clients to better match them with appropriate solutions, as discussed in Chapter 4. Therapists track increases and decreases in specific affects and impulses as well. In Boxes 3.1b, 3.2b, and 3.3b this tracking is indicated by intensity ratings on a 5-point scale (e.g., guilt 4/5, urge to harm self 3/5). During a chain analysis therapists may also assess whether a specific emotional or cognitive link was warranted by the facts of the current situation. Alternatively, therapists may wait until they have selected the link for the solution analysis and then make this discrimination.

Theory

The analysis of controlling variables is determined by the application of both behavioral learning theory and Linehan's (1993a) biosocial theory. Learning theory in general teaches therapists to recognize both classically and operantly conditioned responses, and thus encourages therapists to evaluate both the antecedents and consequences of a target behavior. Operant theory particularly directs therapists to analyze the target behavior's function. The biosocial theory further focuses the analysis by suggesting that therapists focus on emotions as controlling variables. The biosocial theory also requires therapists to identify both skills and motivational deficits.

Analyze the Target Behavior's Function

A behavioral or functional analysis, in which the therapist determines the function or purpose of a behavior, is an essential component of many behavioral treatments. A behavior's function depends on the individual's operant conditioning history with the consequences of that behavior. Every behavior has multiple consequences, but not all of the consequences will influence whether the behavior occurs again. A behavioral analysis focuses on identifying the "functional consequences," which refers to those consequences that reinforce the behavior because they serve a function or help the individual to achieve a goal. Thus, identifying a behavior's function requires that the therapist delineate the consequences of an episode and then determine which of the many consequences have a functional relationship with the target behavior. This identification sometimes requires analyses of multiple episodes of a behavior in similar contexts.

Box 3.1b delineates the multiple consequences of Susan's overdose. Her fear and guilt immediately decreased. She then felt woozy and sick. The man in her apartment called the paramedics and then left. The paramedics arrived, administered treatment, and then transported Susan to the hospital. A psychiatric resident assessed her and admitted her to the psychiatric ward. Susan felt less guilt after the admission. Her boyfriend visited and reassured her about their relationship. Susan then experienced less fear and a close connection to him.

Susan's behavioral analysis revealed that only a few of these consequences reinforced the overdosing. The most powerful reinforcements related to the immediate reduction in the affective antecedents of the behavior, namely, guilt and fear. The reduction in guilt following the hospitalization also reinforced the behavior. This determination directed the solution analysis toward finding less harmful ways to manage the affect. Among the more distal consequences, the reduction in fear and sense of connection resulting from the boyfriend's visit and assurances also reinforced the overdosing. Thus, the solution analysis also needed to address these links. Though the other consequences did not reinforce Susan's behavior, they may reinforce the behavior of other clients. For example, the attention from paramedics and speeding along the road with the ambulance sirens screaming reinforced one client's overdosing. Another client might learn that such overdosing effectively rids him or her of an unwanted sexual partner.

Though an individual may consciously intend a behavior to serve a particular function, the behavior may serve other functions as well. Asking clients about their conscious intent at the start of BCAs can focus and

Box 3.2a. Jane's Narrative

Jane had not slept well the previous evening; she had experienced troubling dreams after an argument with her mother. Throughout the day she had felt lingering guilt about the argument, in which she had criticized her mother for what Jane viewed as her mother's unsympathetic stance about a recent disappointment in Jane's life. While watching an evening television program about dieting, Jane began to feel anxious and to scan her body for "fat places." During an advertisement break she went to her room to try on an old pair of jeans to see if she could fit into them yet. The jeans still did not fit. She then scanned herself in the mirror, while her anxiety continued to rise. Jane began to ruminate about the argument with her mother and about how her brother left the family because he was "fed up" with the focus on Jane and her problems. She went to the bathroom and vomited into the toilet. While vomiting, she felt increasingly tired. She then returned to her bedroom where she slept for several hours.

Box 3.2b. BCA of Jane's vomiting

Target: Vomits three times.

Functions of the target: Reduce fear, queasiness, shame, and guilt and increase sense of control.

| **Vulnerability factors** | Poor sleep. |
| | Rumination and guilt about argument with mother. |

Type of link	**Link in chain**
Prompting event	Views television program about dieting.
Affect	Anxiety (2/5).
Action	Scans body.
Environmental event	Views advertisement on television.
Impulse	Urge to check whether jeans fit.
Action	Tries on jeans.
Sensations	Feel and sight of jeans not fitting.
Affect	Fear (3/5).
Sensation	Queasiness.
Cognitions	Thinks, "It's no good. I'll always be fat."
Action	Looks at herself in the mirror, scanning for evidence of "fat places."
Cognitions	Repeatedly labels "fat" areas.

(continued)

Box 3.2b. (*continued*)

Affect	Fear increases (4/5).
Cognition	Thinks, "I'm always going to be fat."
Cognition	Thinks, "I have no control."
Affect	Shame (3/5).
Cognitions	Thinks, "Mom's right. I'm selfish, hopeless, and too focused on myself."
Affect	Guilt (3/5).
Action	Sits on bed with head in her hands.
Cognition	Notices her stomach "spilling out" of the jeans.
Cognitions	Thinks, "See, that just proves I'm out of control. Look at me. Mom was right."
Affect	Shame increases (4/5).
Cognitions	"Replays" the previous day's argument with her mother.
Cognitions	Thinks, "How can I be so critical of Mom? She just tries to help me."
Affect	Guilt (4/5).
Cognition	Thinks, "I owe her everything."
Cognition	Thinks, "Just think of all the trouble I've caused."
Cognitions	Ruminates about past events.
Cognitions	Thinks, "John [her brother] left because of me. He blames me for Mom being so upset."
Affect	Guilt increases (5/5).
Cognitions	Thinks, "I have an unpayable debt to Mom. There's nothing I can do."
Cognition	Thinks, "I should be punished for what I've done."
Impulse	Urge to vomit (4/5).
Action	Goes to the bathroom to vomit.
Target behavior	Vomits spontaneously at the sight of the toilet.
Negative reinforcement	Fear decreases (3/5).
Negative reinforcement	Queasiness decreases.
Positive reinforcement	Thinks, "Now I'm in control."
Negative reinforcement	Shame decreases (3/5).

(*continued*)

Box 3.2b. (*continued*)

Cognition	Thinks, "It's not enough."
Target behavior	Puts fingers down her throat and vomits twice more.
Sensation	Fatigue.
Negative reinforcement	Fear decreases (1/5), shame decreases (1/5).
Cognition	Thinks, "This is the punishment I deserve."
Negative reinforcement	Guilt decreases (1/5).
Action	Returns to the bedroom and goes to sleep.

Later consequences

Sensation	Smells vomit when she awakens.
Cognition	Thinks, "I've screwed-up again."
Affect	Shame (3/5)

enhance the efficiency of the analysis, but therapists must not confuse an inquiry about the conscious intent with an analysis of the target's function. Consequences other than intended consequences frequently control behavior, often outside of an individual's awareness. For example, Susan intended to escape from her emotions by overdosing, and the overdose served this function. She did not intend to experience a strong sense of connection to her boyfriend, but a similar interpersonal consequence across overdoses had become a secondary reinforcer.

Attend to Emotions

As the biosocial theory proposes that target behaviors function primarily to regulate affect, BCAs must attend closely to emotions, their causes, and their effects. The behavioral analysis clarifies which emotions the target behavior regulates and thus which emotions the therapist must teach the client to manage with other solutions. Several key principles guide the assessment of emotional links.

First, therapists identify and label specific, basic emotions (e.g., joy, sadness, anger, fear, disgust, shame, guilt), as opposed to general "feelings" (e.g., bad, upset). Research by emotions experts supports this emphasis on teaching clients to describe and differentiate discrete emotions. Within the general population, research (Lieberman et al., 2007) has demonstrated that simply selecting an emotion label to describe an emotional expression can reduce amygdala activity. Furthermore, individuals who differentiate more when labeling negative affect appear to use emotion regulation techniques more frequently as well (Barrett, Gross, Christensen, & Benvenuto, 2001). Of particular relevance to DBT targets, a study of underage social drinkers (Kashdan, Ferssizidis, Collins, & Muraven, 2010) found that during periods of intense negative emotions those participants with low emotion differentiation scores drank significantly more than those with high scores, and a study of depression (Demiralp et al., 2012) found participants with major depressive disorder had significantly fewer differentiated negative emotions, independent of emotional intensity.

Understanding and assessing the components of emotions, as described by Linehan (1993a, 1993b, 2014) and in Chapter 1, assists therapists in correctly identifying emotions when clients lack an emotion label for their "feelings" or experience. Furthermore, assessing the emotion components may reveal additional or more specific controlling variables. For example, when Jane identified the emotions that she had experienced before vomiting (see Box 3.2b), her therapist assessed for corresponding sensations, facial expressions, and body posture. Of most importance, Jane felt queasiness as a component of her anxiety, and the immediate decrease in this sensation after vomiting reinforced the target behavior.

Next, therapists monitor changes in the intensity of the emotions throughout the chain. Tracking variations in the intensity assists therapists in identifying those links that influence the emotions and which links the emotions influence. Therapists especially attend to the events, sensations, thoughts, and actions immediately preceding an increase in an emotion's intensity as these variables are likely candidates for controlling the emotion. Equally, therapists assess whether an increase in an emotion's intensity controls the variables that immediately follow, especially any increase in target urges. Operant conditioning theory, however, reminds therapists that the causal relationship may work in the opposite direction. For instance, a decrease in an emotion's intensity may actually control the likelihood of the target behavior immediately preceding the emotion's change. Of course, therapists should not assume that just because two links have chronological proximity that they must have a causal relationship. In particular, when thoughts immediately precede emotions, those thoughts may simply be epiphenomena rather than the cause of the emotion.

In Jane's case, the BCA identified several important links that exacerbated Jane's fear, namely, the sensations associated with nonfitting jeans, labeling fat areas, and thinking that she had no control. The analysis also identified that fear precipitated two critical links—namely, queasiness and self-invalidating cognitions—and that a decrease in fear had a reinforcing relationship with the vomiting that preceded it. Furthermore, the BCA identified negative self-judgments, self-invalidating, and self-blaming thoughts as the primary controlling variables for guilt and shame. In a painful cycle, guilt and shame then controlled these cognitions. The analysis also revealed that as with fear, a decrease in guilt and shame had a reinforcing relationship with the vomiting that preceded it. This relationship, however, depended on the intervening cognition about punishment.

Finally therapists assess for both automatic, direct emotional responses and cognitively mediated emotional responses. Therapists distinguish between automatically elicited emotions (such as biologically based evolutionarily adaptive responses or classically conditioned emotional responses derived from clients' learning histories) and emotions that follow from a cognitive assumption or interpretation about an environmental or an internal event. In contrast to standard cognitive therapy for depression, which tends to emphasize cognitively mediated affect, DBT attends equally to both types of emotional responses. For example, in Jane's case the sensations of nonfitting jeans directly elicited fear, without any intervening thoughts, whereas the guilt and shame depended on the preceding thoughts.

Identify Motivational and Capability Deficits

DBT's biosocial theory states that clients' target behaviors result from a combination of capability deficits and motivational problems, with the latter deriving from clients' classically and operantly conditioned responses. In each BCA, therapists discern those aspects of clients' responses that result from capability versus motivational deficits in order to more accurately guide the solution analysis. For example, Jane's BCA revealed skills deficits in emotion regulation—specifically the capacity to decrease fear, guilt, and shame—and in mindfulness, as she failed to disengage from ruminative, self-validating, judgmental thinking about her history and her body. In terms of motivational problems, the effectiveness of vomiting in decreasing fear, guilt, and shame significantly increased Jane's motivation to vomit through the process of operant conditioning. The rapidity and ease with which Jane vomited indicated a classically conditioned response to viewing the toilet that further weighted Jane's motivation toward vomiting.

Strategies for Efficient and Effective BCAs

Several strategies enhance the efficiency and effectiveness of conducting a BCA. Therapists use these strategies to gain insight into the causal relationships among the links and the function of the target behavior. These strategies include highlighting, recognizing patterns, and generating hypotheses, with highlighting forming the foundation for the other two strategies. During a BCA, highlighting involves calling a client's attention to possibly important links or relationships between links with statements and questions, such as "Your anger seems important," "Did you notice that you became judgmental?" and "It may be relevant that your anger increased after you became judgmental." The first opportunity for therapists to highlight potentially relevant links occurs during the diary card review. A therapist may also highlight aspects of a client's in-session behavior, especially if the in-session behavior relates to a target behavior. For example, during their analysis of Susan's overdose, the therapist observed, "Susan, I noticed that when I mentioned having sex with the man, you hid your face from me and curled up in the chair." Sometimes highlighting alone will suffice to change the in-session behavior. At other times highlighting forms the entry into either a mini-chain and solution analysis of the in-session behavior or an immediate rehearsal of solutions for previously analyzed behaviors.

Over multiple BCAs, DBT therapists recognize repetitive patterns of emotions, cognitions, and actions in the sequence leading to and following from different episodes of the same target and even episodes of different targets. Simple highlighting can then transform into pattern recognition. The examples in the preceding paragraph might become "Have you noticed that judgmental thoughts always precede your anger?" and "Susan, I noticed that whenever you feel shame about what you've done, you hide your face and curl up in the chair while describing it." The patterns may constitute one of the secondary targets described by Linehan (1993a) or be an idiosyncratic pattern for a specific client. For example, Rita demonstrates "active passivity," which Linehan describes as not trying to solve problems for oneself but actively seeking help from others. Rita complained to her psychiatrist about her therapist's "bullying behavior," but did not raise the problem with the therapist directly. Jane's therapist recognized an idiosyncratic pattern in which guilt commonly followed fear or anxiety in a number of chain analyses. When the fear centered on her body image and the guilt resulted from her perceived lack of self-control, Jane was most likely to binge or vomit. When the fear or anxiety related to her college course or spending time with friends and the guilt resulted from her beliefs about not being "a good enough" college student or friend then she was most likely to cut herself. Developing the capacity to reduce and tolerate anxiety, fear, and guilt proved central to treating both of these targets successfully. A therapist's awareness of repeated links or relationships between links can make the therapeutic task more efficient in at least two ways. First, using pattern recognition to postulate potential missing links during a BCA can notably reduce the time required for the BCA. Second, focusing solution analyses on links that occur across contexts or targets may enhance the generalization of solutions.

To maximize therapeutic gains for minimal therapeutic effort, DBT therapists establish which links in the behavioral chain act as controlling or causal variables for the target behavior and other important links. Identifying the causal links requires that therapists generate hypotheses about relationships among the target behavior, its antecedents, and its consequences. Therapists base their hypotheses on the theories underpinning the treatment, namely, the biosocial theory and learning theory. Though both of these theories propose processes through which target behaviors may have initially developed, therapists explain the behavior in terms of current variables rather than historical ones.

As in most cognitive-behavioral treatments, therapists express hypotheses as tentative explanations requiring investigation. For example, a therapist might ask, "Do you think that your judgmental thoughts exacerbate your anger?" or say, "Susan, I'm wondering if you're hiding your face and curling up in the chair because you feel ashamed." Therapists remain aware that their hypotheses may reflect their own theoretical or personal bias rather than reality. They also equally respect clients' hypotheses as potentially valid. Though the therapy strongly encourages clients to comment on therapists' hypotheses and to generate their own, early in therapy, clients may be so bemused by their own experiences that they remain unsure about the accuracy of their therapists' hypotheses and struggle to generate alternative explanations. In the absence of certainty about a hypothesis, the therapist generates solutions based on the best available hypothesis. Implementing the corresponding solutions may confirm the accuracy of the hypothesis, or at least part of it. Alternatively, it may disconfirm the hypothesis, but reveal new information that produces more effective hypotheses. Thus, therapists dialectically synthesize pursuing "the truth" and tolerating uncertainty about "the truth" by intervening despite uncertainty and then learning from the intervention. This attitude of nonattachment to "the truth" of hypotheses exemplifies the dialectical philosophy of the treatment and decreases conflict between clients and therapists about the causal variables leading to target behaviors.

COMMON PROBLEMS

Although the various elements of conducting a BCA aim to increase the efficiency and effectiveness of the analysis, they also multiply the number of ways in which the analysis can go awry. This section addresses common problematic behaviors that therapists can engage in when conducting BCAs. Problems can arise with the structural elements, the theoretical principles, and the strategic points discussed earlier. Problems also occur if therapists fail to treat clients' TIBs that impede BCAs.

Structure

Spending Too Little or Too Much Time on the BCA

Therapists often spend too little or too much time conducting BCAs. The former produces an inadequate or inaccurate analysis of the controlling variables, and the latter leaves insufficient time for the solution analysis. Reasons for insufficient BCAs include misunderstanding what a BCA requires and substituting a client's written chain for an in-session analysis. Therapists who fail to appreciate the type or degree of detail required in a BCA may speed through a chain by accepting broad statements about feelings rather than identifying specific emotions and cognitions or by considering environmental events as sufficient and neglecting clients' psychological responses to these events. This too broad assessment of the chain limits therapists' ability to analyze it. Reviewing BCAs during consultation team meetings provides an efficient way to identify and correct this problem; role-playing also helps.

Therapists may also produce limited BCAs if they use clients' written chains as substitutes for rather than as aides to conducting a BCA during the session. Having clients write their own chains provides therapists with useful overviews of chains and helps therapists to efficiently decide where to focus the analysis. It also may increase clients' ability to recognize the variables that cause or mediate their behavior. Only near the end of treatment, and not always then, will clients have developed sufficient expertise for their own analyses to function effectively in lieu of an analysis with the therapist. Therapists tend to use clients' chains as substitutes either because they fail to notice anything missing or because they worry that not doing so will invalidate clients' efforts. Reviewing clients' chain analyses with the consultation team may help in the first situation. With respect to the latter, further assessing the links and any associated hypotheses identified by the client can both improve the quality of the client's BCA analysis and maximally reinforce the client's contributions to the process.

More often, therapists spend too much, rather than too little, time on the BCA, resulting in insufficient time to generate and implement solutions. This occurs if therapists aim for a "perfect" chain analysis in which they have assessed every minute. Though BCAs do require clarity and precision, they do not require perfection. Therapists who previously learned insight-based models may prolong BCAs because these analyses provide most of the insight during the session. In either circumstance, therapists often benefit from reminding themselves that BCAs serve primarily as the handmaiden to solution analyses. A BCA without a corresponding solution analysis usually proves pointlessly painful. Other therapists continue with the chain analysis because they want to avoid the solution analysis because they have no solutions to offer the client, they do not know how to implement the solutions, or because the client engages in more TIBs during the solution analysis.

Eliciting Mostly Just a Narrative

If simply asked what led to their target behavior, many clients spontaneously provide a narrative of the day's or the week's events. One can understand this response, especially in new clients, as this seems a more socially normative response and many individuals experience such storytelling as validating. Furthermore, many clients have had previous treatments that have reinforced this response. The narrative becomes a problem, however, if the therapist accepts it in lieu of a BCA. This acceptance may result from misunderstanding the structural requirements of a BCA, from engaging in habits learned in another therapy model, or from becoming concerned about the effects of blocking the narrative.

Eliciting a lengthy narrative most commonly occurs when therapists ask unfocused questions. For example, instead of asking for the diary card or while mindlessly reviewing the diary card, some therapists have begun sessions by asking, "How was your week?" After identifying an episode of the target behavior that occurred on a particular day, some therapists have said, "So, tell me about Tuesday." Both of these openers provide the client with a cue for a narrative rather than a chain analysis. Therapists minimize the opportunity for narratives by asking questions that focus the client on the target and its proximate links.

After selecting and defining the target for the session, therapists often anchor themselves in the BCA by establishing the immediate context of the target, including the time when and the location where the target occurred. Therapists may then assess backward from the target to avoid starting too early in the day. Alternatively, they may jump back by asking, "When did the urge first start?" or "When did the urge increase above its baseline?" The chain analysis can then progress forward if the urge started not too long before. Of course, therapists can also teach clients what they mean by "prompting event" and ask about it directly or ask clients to provide a very brief summary of "what happened" and then select a prompting event from this summary. Sometimes therapists ask clients to write a chain before the session and then use it as a tool for starting the in-session BCA. Before starting the BCA, many therapists ask for the clients' best assessment of the target behavior's functions and then use this information to start the chain. For example, if the behavior functioned to decrease anger, the therapist might start the chain by asking what event prompted the anger.

When clients decided to engage in a target behavior early in a day but did not act on the decision until later, therapists sometimes become entangled in the day's events. Therapists have a couple of options in this circumstance. First, they may simply analyze the links immediately preceding and following the target behavior itself, starting with the prompting event for deciding to follow through with the earlier plan. The decision earlier in the day may have made the client more vulnerable to action later, but need not have directly caused it. Many people frequently decide to do something at a later time, but then do not do it (e.g., deciding in the morning to exercise after work, deciding today to clean the house tomorrow, deciding in the evening to rise early to write about BCAs). Alternatively, therapists may analyze the early period between the prompting event and the immediate consequences of the initial decision to harm and the later period when the client acted. Deciding which of these approaches to follow depends on the length of the respective chains and the time required for a solution analysis.

Some therapists allow clients to continue with a narrative because they have judgments or worries about blocking clients from telling their "story" or because they have suffered aversive consequences when they have tried to redirect clients toward a BCA. Some therapists judge themselves as impolite or disrespectful because such blocking violates "normal" rules of social or therapeutic interactions. In a sense, the blocking of storytelling does violate social norms, just as asking someone to remove his or her clothes does, but just as physicians cannot do their jobs without the latter, DBT therapists cannot do their jobs without the former. DBT is neither a social interaction nor a therapy that bases interventions on clients relaying their "stories." In addition to mindfully letting go of any judgments, some cognitive restructuring may assist therapists who have these thoughts. For example, if simply relating a narrative of their experiences significantly improved clients' lives, they probably would not need DBT. If a therapist instead worries that the client might have similar judgments or interpretations, then the therapist can solve the problem by assessing the client's thoughts and orienting the client to reasons for an analysis rather than a story. Usually, therapists provide this orientation during pretreatment and ensure that clients have experienced such an analysis before they commit to the treatment. By orienting and obtaining a commitment from the client, the therapist possesses an agreement to interrupt the client in full narrative flow and return to a chain analysis. Unfortunately, orientation and agreement alone do not always prevent clients from trying to tell their story. In such cases, therapists will need a more comprehensive analysis of the client's TIB and a broader selection of solutions to treat it. Crucially, therapists must understand the function of the storytelling. For example, one client experienced the behavior as very validating. As part of the solution, the therapist expressed more validation when the client focused on the analysis and as little validation as possible when the client became absorbed in a narrative. Also, they agreed that the client could have 5 minutes at the beginning of the session to summarize the situation in her own way and that she could talk about anything after they had completed the behavioral chain and solution analyses for the session.

Focusing Mostly on Vulnerabilities

Therapists sometimes become entangled in dissecting vulnerability factors for the target behavior. Though therapists may address these factors as part of the solution analysis, many vulnerability factors prove either unnecessary or very difficult to change. Therefore, focusing the chain analysis mostly on vulnerabilities usually provides a poor return for the investment. In Susan's overdose following her episode of sex with a stranger (see Box 3.1b), her therapist initially thought about further analyzing the more distal conflict with the boyfriend and the decision to go drinking. She focused the analysis on the period from the prompting event through the consequences, however, because she realized that neither the conflict nor the drinking had elicited any urges to overdose or the emotions directly related to the overdose. Susan had frequently argued with her boyfriend and gone drinking without overdosing, so stopping the target from reoccurring did not require preventing those vulnerabilities. Furthermore, the drinking seemed a rather intransigent problem at this point in treatment and removing all arguments from a relationship seems an unachievable goal. Addressing these issues may have decreased her vulnerability but would not have assisted Susan in solving the complex psychological events that link her sexual behavior with overdosing and its function. Effective DBT therapists focus their analyses more on the most proximate causal variables rather than on multiple, distal vulnerability factors.

Failing to Assess for Urges or Affect or to Track Changes in Their Intensity

A BCA may prove inadequate not because the therapist spent too little time on it, but because the therapist failed to assess for key variables. To generate the best hypotheses about the causal relationship between the links in the chain and the target behavior, therapists need to know which links precipitated impulses or urges to engage in the behavior and which links precipitated increases in the urges. For example, Susan's therapist could hypothesize early in the analysis that the overdosing might function to reduce guilt because she soon learned that strong guilt had immediately preceded the initial self-harm urge. Without this information, the target behavior may appear to have happened more impulsively than it did (e.g., that going to the bathroom suddenly prompted Susan's overdose) and the solution analysis may appear to have fewer opportunities for changing the behavior. Similarly, to generate hypotheses based on the biosocial theory, therapists need to assess for emotions or affective links and changes in their intensity. An absence of information about affect generally causes therapists to miss the primary function of the behavior and makes them more vulnerable to overestimating the impact of interpersonal consequences. If Susan's therapist had not assessed for emotions, she would have missed the primary functions of overdosing and may have assumed that Susan overdosed just to gain reassurance from the boyfriend. Fortunately, this set of problems seems easily corrected if the consultation team reviews therapists' chain analyses for missing impulses and emotions, highlights any such patterns, and then continues to review the analyses of any therapist who consistently misses links until that therapist has corrected the problem.

Organizing Links by Type Rather Than by Chronology

Similar to the problem of not tracking changes in impulses or emotions, therapists sometimes assess links by the type of link, grouping all links of the same type together, rather than assess the links in the order that they occurred. Assessing links by type rather than by chronology interferes with the analysis because it misses information relevant to establishing causality. For example, one therapist initially presented a "chain analysis" that listed vulnerabilities, then all of the affective links together, and then all of the cognitions together. The affective links appeared as "Emotions—happy, angry, embarrassed." This suggests that the client might have felt angry about feeling happy or that she might have felt embarrassed about feeling and expressing anger. In this case, however, the emotions had no causal relationship with one another. Instead, each emotion occurred because of what happened just moments before it. Fortunately, consultation teams also can solve this problem with relative ease by reviewing therapists' chain analyses.

Failing to Differentiate Emotions and Cognitions

Maximally effective solution analyses require therapists to correctly elucidate different types of links as each type of link has a different set of solutions. Unfortunately, therapists frequently fail to differentiate emotions and cognitions because of the way that language occludes the distinction. In everyday language, people alternately use the term "feeling" as a synonym for emotions or sensations and as a referent to any internal experience, such as "My feeling is that she doesn't like me" and "I feel that was stupid." If therapists conceptualize in the vernacular themselves or rely on this language with clients, they risk collecting a set of "feelings" that are an unclear mix of internal experiences, including poorly defined emotion–thought compounds. For example, many therapists accept "I feel hopeless" as a description of an emotion, when actually the statement generally summarizes clients' hopeless thinking. The emotions associated with hopeless thoughts vary across clients. Failing to separate emotions and cognitions leads therapists to insufficiently specify or inaccurately identify controlling variables and hence to overgeneral or inaccurate solutions (i.e., specifying a cognitive solution for an emotional link or vice versa). For example, one therapist accepted "feel hopeless" as an emotion and thus did not bother to assess for any other emotions. Then in the solution analysis he challenged the hopelessness with cognitive techniques, but failed to suggest any emotion-based solutions because he had not actually identified an emotion. Therapists can reduce the likelihood of emotion–cognition confusion by replacing questions about feelings or general statements, such as "Tell me more about it," with specific questions about emotions and thoughts. Even without this prompt, however, clients will still use the term "feeling" in a variety of ways and will mislabel cognitions as emotions. Clients' use of "feeling" serves as one cue to the possibility of confusion. Also, when clients label an experience as an emotion, comparing that experience with a mental list of the basic emotions helps to detect mislabeling. In such instances, therapists then help clients to differentiate the emotions from the cognitions. For example, one client frequently said she "felt abandoned" during the analyses. The therapist determined that "felt abandoned" was actually a thought and then assessed for related thoughts and emotions. The chain revealed, in sequence, the thought "They abandoned me," the thought "I can't cope," followed by the emotion of fear and the thought "They shouldn't have done that," followed by the emotion of anger.

Theory

Applying Another Theoretical Model to the Analysis

Therapists who learned nonbehavioral theories before learning DBT often struggle to inhibit the application of those theoretical models when they analyze the behaviors of DBT clients. For example, some nonadherent DBT therapists try to explain clients' behaviors in terms of clients' distant pasts, rather than in terms of the current controlling variables. Though an adherent DBT therapist might suggest that an adult client had taken heroin because he started to panic when he had flashbacks of being sexually abused and the heroin effectively reduced the flashbacks and panic, the therapist would not suggest that the client took the heroin simply because he suffered sexual abuse as a child. Though some clients might experience the focus on their pasts as more validating, such a focus usually delays solving clients' current problems. Some therapists tend to apply a model that encourages them to search for a single, key controlling variable, such as a core cognition, rather than for multiple controlling variables. This focus significantly restricts the options during the solution analysis.

Applying another theoretical model can result from either a knowledge deficit about DBT theoretical principles or from motivational issues. In the former situation, the consultation team might solve the problem by providing more didactic information about the principles, role-playing the application of the principles in an analysis, assigning the therapist relevant homework or regularly reviewing the therapist's BCAs. When the latter situation arises, the consultation team may need to conduct a brief behavioral analysis of the therapist's behavior to identify the motivational factors that control the TIB and then generate corresponding solutions. For example, one therapist persisted in basing her understanding of her client's behavior on the client's childhood abuse. An analysis of this TIB revealed that the therapist had a strong attachment to the belief that the behaviors of clients with BPD occurred because of their abuse history. When she even slightly attempted to challenge this belief, she began to doubt her past clinical work in other models, and then she experienced fear, followed by guilt. Despite all of this, she still wanted to do DBT, so together with the team, she developed a set of solutions that included mindfulness and cognitive restructuring for her doubt, a variety of solutions for the emotions, and another analysis from the team as an aversive consequence if the TIB reoccurred.

Simplifying Motivation as "Want" or "Will"

In assessing the reasons for the presence or absence of a behavior, therapists sometimes confuse the behavioral concept of motivation with the common concepts of either "want" or "will." A therapist, therefore, may conceptualize a motivational problem simply as a client "wanting" to engage in a target behavior or "not wanting" to engage in a skillful behavior. Many clients give oversimplified explanations of their motivation to therapists because they have been raised in invalidating environments that oversimplify how to change behavior and instead emphasize willpower (see Chapter 1). Even therapists who generally know the difference between will and motivation may begin to confuse them if the client does. As highlighted in Chapter 1, behavioral treatments have a more comprehensive understanding of motivation, in which neither "want" nor "will" have a starring role. Indeed, clients often engage in target behaviors that they really do not "want" to do or that they "found" themselves doing without ever deciding to do. Numerous factors, including emotional and environmental antecedents and contingencies, as well as cognitions, impinge on the likelihood of emitting any given behavior. In assessing for the controlling variables of target behaviors, therapists broaden their understanding of motivation to encompass all of these aspects. In Rita's case, her anxiety, anger, and learning history of threats that reduced environmental demands have all impacted her motivation to threaten rather than use her few, frail interpersonal skills to express her worries to her treatment team.

Though "want to" or "don't want to" may simply reflect a client's motivational statement, the cognition itself may directly impact the motivation to engage in the behavior. Fortunately, behavioral change remains possible without changing the "want" or the "will." For example, one client needed to exercise more because of severe medical problems and so agreed to analyze episodes of not doing her exercise. When the therapist first analyzed an episode, the client simply said, "I didn't want to exercise, so I decided not to do it." Sharing the client's understanding of motivation, the therapist simply accepted the client's volitional analysis and then focused on increasing the client's desire to exercise, primarily by highlighting the negative consequences of not exercising and the positive consequences of exercising. Not surprisingly, this solution did not increase the client's exercising at all. After consultation from the team, the therapist conducted a comprehensive BCA and discovered a number of variables that influenced the client's motivation to exercise, including some that actually punished her exercising. The solution analysis broadened significantly to address these other factors. Of particular interest, the client revealed that before starting exercise she frequently asked herself the question, "Do I want to exercise?" and most often answered, "No!" Asking and answering the question in this way further decreased her motivation to exercise. The therapist coached the client on mindfully describing "don't want to" as a thought, letting the thought go and then starting to exercise. When the client implemented mindfulness and the other solutions, she increased the frequency of exercising, even though she still never "wanted" to exercise.

In another case, an adolescent client who had battled with urges to self-harm for several hours stated during the BCA that when she had showered she had just cut herself "in the end" because she had wanted to do it and "was fed up" with using her skills. The therapist accepted this explanation and proceeded to offer solutions for what he viewed as the client's "willfulness." Following consultation with a DBT supervisor, the next time the behavior occurred the therapist more closely analyzed the events around cutting in the shower. He discovered that simply entering the shower, even without existing urges to cut, triggered urges to cut because of a classically conditioned association between cutting and the shower. Also, for this client taking a *hot* shower further increased her emotional arousal and tension, which then further fueled her urges to cut. The new solution analysis added showering at lower temperatures, especially if she already had urges, treating the classically conditioned response, and developing new associations among showering and pampering and self-soothing. Solutions for willfulness formed no part in the effective solution analysis for the behavior!

Not Assessing Function Accurately

In their analysis of the consequences of a target behavior, therapists may fail to identify any function(s) at all or fail to specify the function(s) accurately. Failing to identify any function at all usually occurs when therapists have forgotten that the "behavioral" in a BCA equals a functional analysis. In addition to remembering this essential principle, many therapists prevent the problem by routinely, though briefly, assessing for the function before starting the chain analysis. Reasons for failing to specify the function accurately include identifying only a general, vague function, confusing function with consequences and confusing function with conscious intent. As an example of the first reason, one therapist had a client who vomited to "feel better." The therapist initially accepted this vague function, but then realized that the solution analysis seemed too generalized and too focused on "cheering" the client. The therapist then identified the more specific functions of reducing shame and increasing a perception of self-control. With this more specific information, the therapist developed a more effective solution analysis by generating solutions that more accurately matched these functions.

With respect to confusing functions and consequences, therapists sometimes automatically list all of the target behavior's consequences as functions, without assessing whether each consequence actually reinforced the behavior. In Boxes 3.1b, 3.2b, and 3.3b, all of the targets had multiple consequences, but only some related to the functions. In Rita's case, the therapist had previously conducted a behavioral analysis that

---

Box 3.3a. Rita's Narrative

Rita attended a review with the unit psychiatrist. She had been feeling nervous all day about the review as she worried that the psychiatrist would reduce her medication or would suggest more home leave that she did not want yet. She also received a phone call from her father who slammed the phone down saying that she was a hopeless case when he discovered that she was in the hospital "again!" At the start of the review meeting Rita felt more anxious as her case manager was not there and the nurse in the review meeting did not know her well. The psychiatrist began by asking her about her mood and reviewing her symptoms, in particular her recent suicidal thinking and self-harm on the ward. Rita said that she thought that nobody understood her, that her therapist "bullied" her by constantly asking difficult questions, and that she wanted to make a complaint about the therapist and change therapies. The psychiatrist then ended the meeting.

Box 3.3b. BCA of Rita's Threatening

Target: Threatens to file a formal complaint that her individual therapist is "bullying" her by focusing on stopping self-harm and suggesting that she use skills as solutions.

Function of the target: Decrease anxiety and obtain "validation" from the environment about her distress and her difficulties.

Vulnerability factors	Invalidating phone call from father.
	Case manager absent.
	Anxious throughout the day about outcome of meeting.

Type of link	**Link in chain**
Prompting event	Psychiatrist says, "I notice that you have self-harmed three times recently on the unit. I'm wondering how you feel things are going here?"
Affect	Anxiety (3/5).
Impulse	Urge to leave (3/5).
Cognition	Thinks, "He thinks I'm getting worse, that I don't deserve to be here."
Affect	Anxiety increases (5/5)
Cognition	Thinks, "I'm working as hard as I can."
Cognition	Thinks, "They don't understand how hard I'm working."
Cognition	Thinks, "People never understand me."
Cognition	Thinks, "My team should understand me."
Affect	Anger (3/5).
Action	Says, "I'm working as hard as I can, but nobody understands me. Everyone just keeps pushing and pushing."
Affect	Anger (4/5).
Environmental event	Psychiatrist says, "I'm sure people do realize that it's difficult."
Affect	Anger (5/5).
Action	Says, "No, they don't. My therapist just keeps telling me to stop harming and to use skills, skills, skills. What the f**k does she know?"

(continued)

Box 3.3b. (*continued*)

Target behavior	Says, "I'm going to complain about her bullying me. You all bully me. I'll complain to the hospital managers about the lot of you."
Negative reinforcement	Anxiety decreases (4/5).
Environmental event	Psychiatrist says, "This is obviously all a bit difficult for you today. Maybe we should end now," and then ends the meeting.
Negative reinforcement	Anxiety decreases (2/5).
Environmental event	Nurse offers her an as-needed medication and a warm drink.
Positive reinforcement	The nurse tells her that the psychiatrist is "very concerned" about her and asks if she understands the complaints procedure.
Cognition	Thinks, "They understand how difficult it is for me now."
Negative reinforcement	Anxiety decreases (0/5).
Emotion	Anger decreases (0/5).

had a similarly complex web of emotional, cognitive, and interpersonal consequences. Having carefully tracked the different types of emotions and changes in their intensity throughout the chain, the therapist initially assumed that the decrease in anger indicated that the threatening functioned to reduce anger as well as anxiety, but this assumption proved faulty. Similarly, the therapist had assumed that the time with the nurse and the offer of a drink and medication also reinforced the threatening, but again the therapist had assumed incorrectly. For Rita, the only aspect of the interaction with the nurse that reinforced her behavior was the nurse's communication of the psychiatrist's concern. As clients often have some awareness of their behaviors' functions, discussing potential functions with the client helps to differentiate functional from incidental consequences. Noticing patterns across behavioral analyses and whether changing certain consequences decreases the frequency of the target also helps to extract the functions from the consequences.

With respect to confusing functions and conscious intent, therapists sometimes simply substitute clients' statements of conscious intent for functional analyses. Though a statement of intent usually captures a target's primary function, the statement can prove insufficiently specific or inaccurate in identifying the function. For example, when asked directly about the intent of suicide attempts, many clients respond with "I wanted to die." In such cases, "wanting to die" does describe the intent, but usually not the specific function. (Of course, if "wanting to die" is the only function, the therapist reaches a blind alley as the therapy cannot focus on finding alternative methods to die!) In these circumstances, therapists must pursue the analysis by asking what dying would accomplish. Most clients answer by saying that death would stop or relieve their pain, suffering, or some other aversive experience. As "pain" and "suffering" still lack sufficient specificity, therapists would continue the assessment to determine which specific emotions, thoughts, sensations, or situations the client wants to end. The behavioral analysis requires refinement until the therapist has a function that the solution analysis can treat. For example, one session progressed only haltingly when the therapist initially accepted the client's stated desire of being dead as the function of her overdose. When the therapist finally asked about the purpose of dying, the client stated that she wanted to be with her dead mother, leaving the therapist with no viable solutions. After coaching from the consultation team, the next time an overdose occurred, the therapist pursued the behavioral analysis further by asking about the function of being with her mother. When the client responded that she wanted to stop "feeling bad," the therapist asked for clarification of feeling "bad." They finally determined that the client wanted to decrease her sense of loneliness and that even just planning an overdose achieved this by increasing her sense of connection to her mother. The solution analysis then focused on alternative means of achieving this function, with the additional solution of challenging the client's certainty that she would join her mother if she committed suicide.

As another example of confusing intent and function, some clients state that they wanted "to punish" themselves. In behavioral terms, this is a nonsequitur as only behavior can be punished. The therapist and client must define more precisely which actions the client aims to punish. For example, a client might intend that a consequence like cutting will punish his or her assaultive actions earlier in the day. Usually, however, the target behavior has no impact on the repetition of any earlier actions. Instead, thinking of the target behavior as punishment often contributes to the reinforcement of the target behavior. Jane's behavioral analysis (see Box 3.2b) demonstrates this phenomenon. Jane's belief that she administered the punishment that she thought she deserved contributed to the reinforcement of her vomiting behavior because it largely controlled the decrease in guilt. This decrease in guilt then motivated Jane to maintain the dysfunctional belief. Clarifying the technical definitions of reinforcement and punishment and reviewing the relative merits of punishment as a change strategy can encourage clients to change dysfunctional beliefs about punishment. If punishment seemed an appropriate solution, the therapist and client could devise less harmful and more helpful punishing consequences, such as implementing reparations. For some clients, however, the belief has such a strong function itself that therapists must try to prevent reinforcement of the belief. For example, Jane's therapist tried to minimize the reduction in guilt by emphasizing that Jane had neither done anything to repair the damage to her family nor anything to prevent similar behavior in the future, thus the guilt remained as warranted as before she vomited.

Strategies

Failing to Highlight Unmindful Thinking

Therapists frequently fail to highlight clients' unmindful thinking, even when the thinking contributes to target behaviors. Therapists may miss unmindful thinking when it occurs as part of the BCA, but they seem even more likely not to highlight it when it occurs during a session. As clients often express the same unmindful thoughts in sessions that cause problems out of sessions, missing the thought in session may mean missing the best opportunity to help clients to notice it. The failure to highlight unmindful thinking tends to result from therapists either misunderstanding what mindfulness entails, not mindfully attending to clients' cognitive processes, or becoming inhibited by concerns about how clients will respond to the highlighting.

In contrast to other mindfulness-based therapies, DBT teaches mindfulness in the skills training group by engaging clients in a variety of brief mindfulness exercises. For inexperienced practitioners of mindfulness, this can result in confusion between mindfulness exercises, which provide opportunities to shape the skill of mindfulness, and *being* mindful. Being mindful involves viewing reality as it is in the current moment and letting go of thoughts that obstruct this view. To help clients accomplish this, therapists need to develop and maintain an awareness of their clients' patterns of unmindful thinking. This section highlights two of the most universally common types of unmindful thinking (in Western culture, at least), namely, judgmental thinking and making assumptions.

Judgmental thinking is often the most easily recognized type of unmindful thinking, as certain words such as "bad," "wrong," "should," "shouldn't," "too," and "deserve" often alert therapists to possible judgmental thoughts. In Jane's case, her therapist easily noticed the "should" in "I should be punished for what I've done" and the "too" in "I'm selfish, hopeless, and too focused on myself." Therapists must remain cautious not only about noticing thoughts that contain these cues but also about automatically assuming that these words alone indicate judgmental thinking. For example, people often use "should" conditionally (e.g., "I should exercise more if I want to become fitter"), rather than judgmentally. The use of other terms with a "negative connotation," such as Jane is "selfish," usually indicate a judgment, but not always. For example, "I'm fat" may express a judgmental thought if the individual thinks of fat as a failing, but it may only describe a fact about the individual's body fat percentage.

Individuals also frequently make a wide variety of assumptions, including unmindful interpretations about the causes of behavior. In Jane's case, she automatically assumed that she would "always be fat." Rita (see Box 3.3b) immediately interpreted the psychiatrist's comments about her self-harm as indicating that he thought that she did not deserve a place in the unit and that he didn't understand how hard she had worked. Compared with judgments, however, assumptions generally have fewer clear signals of their presence, making them more difficult to detect. For example, one client repeatedly said, "I can't" whenever she tried a new skill and did not immediately succeed. The therapist initially missed identifying the statement as a potential interpretation of why the skill had not succeeded. When the therapist eventually highlighted and investigated the interpretation, the analysis revealed that the client did not succeed because she had not applied the skills for long enough rather than because she lacked the skills. Also, unlike judgments, assumptions may reflect known facts or eventually prove accurate, but by their very definition, assumptions are beliefs without or before any evidence to support them. Rita could have correctly interpreted her psychiatrist's statement, but she could not ascertain the veracity of her beliefs solely on the basis of what he said.

Even if they understand mindfulness, therapists will still fail to highlight unmindful thinking if they do not remain mindful of the clients' thinking during sessions. Sometimes, therapists become caught in the content of clients' thinking rather than attending to the type of thinking. For example, every time one client described herself as a "bad mother," the therapist reacted by challenging the content of the thought rather than labeling the judgmental nature of the thought. The challenging only elicited more proof from the client for her belief and cost the client an opportunity to learn mindfulness. Focusing on the process of cognition rather than content distinguishes DBT from many other

CBTs. At other times, therapists may become generally nonattentive, especially if they have not strengthened their own capacity for mindfulness.

Therapists' capacities to recognize clients' unmindful thinking processes and to remain mindful during sessions will improve as they attend to similar patterns in their own thinking and practice mindfulness. Therapists frequently have unmindful thoughts about their clients, sometimes without awareness. The DBT consultation team assists therapists in recognizing their own unmindful thinking processes. For example, therapists often become frustrated by the relatively slow rate of progress in therapy. This frustration may lead to interpretations that the clients "are resisting change" or assumptions that they "are not trying sufficiently hard" or "are incapable of change." Such unmindful cognitions may elicit more aversive affect and tend to demotivate therapists from working with the client. To treat these cognitive processes, therapists utilize the same skills that they advocate to clients.

Finally, therapists sometimes inhibit highlighting if they have concerns about how clients will respond. If a therapist simply worries about a client's response without any evidence that the client will respond poorly, the therapist can begin to treat the inhibition by sharing the concerns with the client. Like most individuals, clients seldom enjoy having their unmindful thoughts highlighted, but they generally do not object either. If a client does object, the therapist can then address the reasons. For example, when one client assumed that the highlighting occurred because the therapist disliked the client, the therapist simply oriented the client to the actual reasons for highlighting. In another case with the same therapist, the therapist first highlighted the client's interpretation and asked the client to "look for the evidence" and to generate alternative explanations. After the client implemented this cognitive restructuring, the therapist reinforced the client's efforts by orienting the client to the purpose of highlighting. The therapist chose this combination with the second client because that client frequently made erroneous assumptions, whereas the first client did not. In cases where the client's past TIBs justify the therapist's concerns, the client will progress more if the therapist continues to highlight unmindful thinking and then analyzes and treats the behavior when it happens. In one case, the therapist avoided highlighting assumptions because highlighting sometimes resulted in the client shouting at him. With the consultation team's encouragement, the therapist returned to highlighting and analyzed the client's shouting when it occurred. The analysis revealed that the client experienced intense shame whenever the therapist highlighted unmindful cognitions.

The shame prompted immediate anger toward the therapist, and the anger elicited the urge to shout, which functioned to block the repetition of the highlighting and the maintenance of the shame. The solution analysis focused particularly on reducing the intensity of the shame and, dialectically, tolerating low levels of shame.

Relying on Socratic Questioning to Elicit Insight

Overreliance on Socratic questioning to elicit insight often unnecessarily prolongs the chain analysis and may also increase clients' distress during BCAs. Therapists' tendency to rely on Socratic questioning arises for several reasons. First, some therapists worry that making suggestions or hypothesizing about what occurred or why "puts words in the client's mouth" or they worry that inaccurate hypotheses may damage the therapeutic relationship. DBT, however, discourages therapists from treating clients as fragile and encourages mind reading (a type of validation) and sharing hypotheses. Many clients especially benefit from these strategies early in treatment because they never previously learned to label their internal experiences or to assess the causal relationships among their experiences. Most clients do not hesitate to challenge any suggestions that they consider inaccurate. If the therapist genuinely believes that a particular client would not contradict the therapist if he or she disagreed, the therapist might assess the problem (e.g., asking, "You aren't just agreeing with me because I'm the therapist are you?" and then analyzing why if the client answers affirmatively) or might simply offer multiple-choice answers, including "none of the above."

Therapists may also persist with Socratic questioning because of particular beliefs about causal mechanisms. Some therapies propose that insight operates as a primary mechanism of therapeutic change and that the effectiveness of the insight depends on the client, and not the therapist, producing the insight. DBT, however, does not propose insight as a primary mechanism of change. Indeed, the model suggests that insight often proves insufficient and may even prove unnecessary. DBT presumes that changes in target behaviors result primarily from the implementation of effective, new solutions. As long as someone in the therapy room understands the controlling variables for the target behavior, a solution analysis can proceed. Insight by the client may further motivate the client to implement the solutions, but it may not. When clients cannot articulate their inner state, therapists should increase mind reading rather than perseverating with Socratic questions. When clients cannot or do not provide insights into the causal connections among cognitions, affects, impulses, and actions, therapists must generate more hypotheses.

Jumping to Conclusions Rather Than Generating Hypotheses

Although many disciplines share the mantra "always assess, never assume," assuming occurs so frequently in everyday life that, not surprisingly, it happens in therapy as well. Rather than generating hypotheses, therapists sometimes make assumptions or "jump to conclusions" (in the colloquial sense) about various aspects of clients' experiences and behaviors. Though correct assumptions may increase the speed of solving problems, erroneous ones not only decrease the speed, they can also derail the process, sometimes causing the therapy relationship to crash. Assumptions about clients' capability and motivational deficits seem most likely to derail treatment, either by leading therapists to misidentify controlling variables and thus generate a faulty set of solutions or by creating conflict between the therapist and client. If therapists assume that a problematic behavior occurred because of capability deficits, they may miss critical motivational factors, whereas if they assume that motivational factors controlled a behavior, they may miss relevant capability deficits. When therapists jump to the conclusion that external contingencies motivated the behavior, they usually neglect important internal contingencies.

Although therapists might make assumptions about capability deficits for a number of reasons, these assumptions tend to occur most commonly in response to clients' unrecognized assumptions about their own capabilities. More specifically, when clients say that they "couldn't" or "can't" do something, therapists often accept these statements as accurate descriptions of clients' capabilities and fail to further assess the facts. These statements may actually reflect facts about clients' capabilities, but clients often make the automatic assumption about their abilities, confusing "didn't" with "couldn't." Furthermore, many clients use "can't" when they want to avoid doing something, having learned that most people will decrease demands in response. In response to such statements, therapists need to separate the interpretation from the facts and the capability deficits from the motivational factors. For example, one client usually responded to suggested interpersonal solutions (particularly to saying, "No") with "I can't." Initially, the therapist assumed that the client lacked interpersonal skills and so taught the relevant skills. While role playing, the client appeared to have the required skills but still persisted with "I can't." When the therapist analyzed the problem further, the client revealed a fear of how the other person would respond. Without attention to this motivational factor, the client would never have used the interpersonal skills. In a similar case, the "I can't" again did not reflect a skills deficit, but instead resulted from the thought "I don't deserve to get what I want." Increasing the client's appropriate requests required more treatment of the inhibiting cognition than teaching of interpersonal skills.

At other times, therapists jump to the conclusion that motivational factors must have controlled behaviors, neglecting to assess for capability deficits. Therapists become particularly vulnerable to such an error if they underestimate the difficulty of generalizing skills across environmental contexts. The emotional instability of clients with BPD provides a particularly variable intrapersonal context for using new skills. Thus, clients may exhibit skills in one context but fail to emit the same skills in another context. Linehan (1993a) refers to this pattern as "apparent competence." For example, one client skillfully, though too frequently, negotiated changes to psychotherapy session times, but she often wanted to negotiate those changes because of conflicts with medical appointments, which she never asked to change. When therapists observe such differences or other professionals report observations that reflect these differences, therapists sometimes assume that clients have a motivational deficit, rather than first assessing whether the client possesses skills to engage in similar behaviors but in different contexts. The therapist in the case above made such an assumption and therefore focused on contingency management as a solution, but this proved ineffective. To replace assumptions with analysis, the therapist will benefit from first understanding the function of the target behavior and then assessing why the client did not achieve the function in a less problematic way. In addition, asking clients to demonstrate how they did or would implement a particular skill often provides the best means to assess whether they possess that skill in their repertoire.

Because Rita clearly had the capacity to articulate her view that her therapist bullied her and that she wished to change therapists, her therapist assumed that Rita therefore had the capacity to express worries about home leave as well. The therapist then jumped to the conclusion that only motivational factors controlled Rita's threatening. The DBT team highlighted this assumption and encouraged further assessment. When the therapist asked Rita to role-play expressing worries about very basic concerns, they discovered that, in addition to motivational factors, Rita lacked basic skills in articulating anxiety and its related causes in clearly intelligible ways to others.

Even when therapists have correctly assumed that motivational factors controlled clients' behaviors, they sometimes incorrectly assume that interpersonal or other environmental contingencies controlled the behaviors, when actually the behaviors functioned to change clients' emotional or other internal experiences. These faulty assumptions lead problem solving astray and can damage the therapy relationship, as clients experience such errors as emotionally distressing as well as invalidating. These errors often occur when therapists have more information about environmental consequences than internal consequences before they begin the analysis. If the client is an adolescent, has a complex treatment network, or lives in a hospital or prison, the therapist might have received unsolicited but substantial information about the impact of the client's behavior on others before having a chance to speak to the client. Also, if clients' behaviors have direct consequences for therapists, therapists become more vulnerable to jumping to conclusions based on those consequences. For example, when Angie, an inpatient, went absent without leave, her therapist worried intensely about her and spent a lot of time trying to find her. The therapist jumped to the conclusion that Angie had left to attract attention and elicit concern. She then became more angry than worried. During the first therapy session after the police had found and returned Angie to the hospital, the therapist confronted her about leaving the hospital to attract attention, and Angie then immediately "stormed out" of the session. The therapist's DBT team highlighted that the therapist had substituted jumping to conclusions for generating hypotheses about motivational factors and conducting a behavioral analysis. When the therapist met again with Angie, she first profusely apologized for jumping to conclusions and then began a BCA of leaving the hospital. This time Angie remained in the session and revealed that the behavior had functioned to reduce her shame about the hospitalization and to increase her sense of control, factors that the therapist had not considered but that had also controlled her departure from the previous session.

Failing to Treat Clients' TIBs

Therapists frequently encounter client behaviors that disrupt the BCA. TIBs include remaining completely mute; refusing to do the BCA or answer relevant questions; repeatedly and unmindfully saying, "I don't know" or "I can't remember"; answering questions with too much irrelevant information; changing the topic; dissociating; and sobbing intensely. Sometimes a brief intervention, such as labeling the TIB, expressing disapproval, suggesting a skill, or clarifying the consequences of the TIB can stop the behavior without further analysis and enable a quick return to the BCA. For example, in response to Rita's frequent "I don't remember" responses during BCAs, her therapist simply clarified that they could treat the memory problem with an additional detailed daily diary sheet for completion several times a day. Rita responded to this contingency by immediately remembering more. Adjustments to the components of the BCA itself can also reduce the TIB or limit its impact. For example, some clients remember more easily if the therapist assesses the physical context of the target before the psychological links. If a client cannot remember links in the chain due to dissociation immediately preceding the target behavior, the BCA can focus on the antecedents of the dissociation and the links after the dissociation stops. Often, however, TIBs require more extensive treatment involving their own brief behavioral chain and solution analyses. In such cases, therapists still are applying the treatment adherently, as clients can often learn as much from the treatment of their in-session behaviors as from other targets. Adherence problems arise only if the therapist does not apply DBT to the client's TIB and does not return to the original BCA, or otherwise reinforces the client's TIB.

On occasion, therapists fail to treat clients' behaviors that interfere with BCA because they do not recognize the behavior as interfering. For example, a therapist might listen to a client's narrative of the day that self-harm occurred or stories about the distant past because the therapist has not learned the effective parameters of a BCA or becomes interested in the "story" and forgets the analysis. Though therapists may identify this problem themselves, it often becomes apparent only when teams listen to session recordings or analyze another problem that the therapist brought for consultation (e.g., "I never have enough time for a solution analysis"). When the team, rather than the therapist, first notices the problem, the therapist often benefits from closer monitoring of sessions and from team role plays in which the therapist practices noticing the "client's" TIB and then treating it.

More often, a therapist notices that a client's behavior is substantially interfering with the BCA, but fails to treat it successfully. In many instances, therapists decide not to attempt to treat clients' TIBs, despite their persistence. In other instances, therapists attempt to treat the TIBs, but the attempt goes awry. The reasons for not treating clients' TIBs or abandoning attempts to do so seem as diverse as clients' reasons for engaging in them. For example, two therapists had clients who responded frequently with "I don't remember" at the start of BCAs, and both therapists responded by quickly discontinuing the BCAs. One therapist stated that he did not know how else to respond, whereas the other therapist reported that she expected that the client would "feel invalidated and withdraw" if she pushed the client to remember. When two other therapists noticed their clients veering away from doing chain analyses and into talking about the distant past, the therapists both attempted to block the TIBs but abandoned their attempts. One therapist reported that he had stopped because the client quickly became angry when he tried to block her, whereas the other therapist, who tried for a bit longer, said that she "felt like I constantly had to reorient [the client]" and it "took a lot of effort." Previous sections of this chapter have discussed therapists' interfering emotions and cognitions.

Problem Definition and Client Motivation

Many therapists, particularly novices, report that they do not know how to describe clients' TIB effectively. Some therapists manage this deficit by not discussing their clients' TIBs. Other therapists try, but when their description deviates from the facts, clients punish the attempt. In such instances, consultation teams can help therapists apply the principles of behavioral definition as discussed in Chapter 2. Describing the form of the behavior specifically, rather than summarizing, and noticing other aspects of the context can help. Of course, therapists need to separate their description of the behavior from their judgmental thoughts or emotions about the behavior. Crucially, therapists also should refrain from confusing the behavior with its function or making assumptions about the function or links in the chain. For example, a therapist might say, "I've noticed that whenever I ask questions about your emotions or thoughts before you cut, you say, 'I don't know.' Have you noticed that too?" The therapist would not say, "You're trying to avoid doing the BCA," "You've become resistant to treatment," or "You're not committed to doing the treatment." The emphasis on differentiating the behavior and its function does not imply, however, that therapists should not generate hypotheses about the function. Indeed, hypothesis generation can increase session efficiency by decreasing the time required for analysis. In response to "I don't know," for example, a therapist might hypothesize, "When you say, 'I don't know,' I wonder if you think that if you tell me your thoughts or emotions that I'll push you to do something about them, and you hope to avoid that by saying 'I don't know.' Or is it that you simply don't know how to identify your thoughts and emotions and need me to teach you how?"

Sometimes therapists decide not to target clients' TIBs or to abandon targeting because they cannot motivate clients to collaborate with the targeting. Usually, offering to help clients use other solutions that achieve the function of the TIB but with fewer side effects provides a strong motivation. Perhaps one of the most significant errors that therapists make when targeting clients' TIBs, however, is not attending sufficiently to the behavior's function. TIBs related to BCAs generally function to stop BCAs that elicit a negative emotion. As with higher targets, therapists can also motivate clients by linking the treatment of TIBs to clients' intermediate or long-term goals. For example, a client who dissociates during BCAs may agree to treat the in-session behavior if doing so will also decrease dissociation in other contexts. An adolescent client who wanted others to treat her as "mature" had a habit of impulsively leaving therapy sessions when she experienced strong emotions during a BCA. The therapist enhanced the client's motivation to treat this TIB by linking it to her goal of others treating her as "mature." Early in therapy, Susan experienced intense shame about her sexual behavior and engaged in several TIBs to avoid BCAs that involved the sexual behavior. The therapist first validated Susan's urge to avoid as a normative social response to engaging in behavior that violated her values. The therapist then highlighted Susan's goal of changing her pattern of sexual behavior and clarified that they could not achieve this goal if the TIBs continued. She also addressed the function of the TIBs by teaching Susan other ways to regulate and tolerate her shame during BCAs. Essential to increasing motivation to target the behavior, therapists must avoid the error of making assumptions about what will motivate clients. For example, a review of long-term consequences may seem irrelevant to a client who has intense negative emotions during a session, and not all clients care about having more time with or more approval from their therapists.

Solution Analysis

Perhaps the most common reason that therapists report for deciding not to treat clients' TIBs is that they do not know how to solve the problem. Often, if therapists remind themselves to analyze the behavior's controlling variables and then treat those variables as they would other targets, they realize that they do know solutions for the problem. For example, if a therapist determines that a client's intense but unwarranted shame inhibits disclosure during a BCA, the therapist would suggest solutions similar to those used for treating unwarranted shame outside of sessions, particularly exposure, acting opposite to emotions, and mindfulness. If a therapist determines that a client repeatedly says "I don't know" when asked about emotions during a BCA because the client lacks the ability to identify specific emotions, the therapist would then teach the client skills for describing emotions. After implementing solutions for the TIB, the therapist and client then return to the original BCA.

If the client experiences extreme emotional, cognitive, or behavioral dysregulation in session that prevents a collaborative analysis of the TIB, the therapist proceeds directly to a solution analysis focused on re-regulating the client. Usually in these situations, the solution generation relies more on the therapist and requires solutions with less cognitive capacity, and the solution implementation requires more intervention by, or specific instructions from, the therapist. For example, when extreme emotional arousal occurs, therapists first would focus on decreasing the emotion by coaching clients in the application of emotion regulation skills, in particular acting opposite to the current emotional action urges. Rather than simply suggesting acting opposite, however, the therapist would identify each of the client's emotional actions and instruct the client how to act opposite to each action. If a client dissociates, the therapist first would attend to ensuring that the client reassociates, using skills such as grounding techniques, intense sensations, breathing, and some types of mindfulness. Rather than just listing the skills, however, the therapist likely would need to provide continual coaching in how to use the chosen skill(s) until the client reassociates. After the client becomes regulated, the therapist and client can conduct a brief analysis of the TIB so that the BCA of the original target can proceed without disruption and a similar TIB will not derail the session again.

Behavioral Conceptualization

Frequently, a therapist may attempt to treat a client's TIB, but without thoroughly applying a behavioral formulation to resolve the problem. The lack of behavioral formulation can cause therapists to try solutions that do not match the problem, to implement solutions insufficiently, or even to implement solutions that reinforce the client's TIB. For example, therapists sometimes implement solutions for clients' TIBs without any assessment of, or even hypotheses about, the function of the TIB or other controlling variables. One therapist tended to respond automatically to a client's noncollaborative behaviors only by highlighting the negative consequences of that behavior on their relationship. When she complained to the team that the client's TIBs persisted, the team highlighted two problems with the solution analysis. First, the therapist had only assumed but never assessed whether the client experienced harming the relationship as a punishing consequence, and second, the solution analysis relied on a potentially punishing consequence rather than analyzing and treating the key controlling variables of the noncollaborative behavior. Occasionally, when solution implementation does not yield immediate results, therapists abandon the solution too quickly. Though persisting with an ineffective solution makes no sense, some solutions do require more persistence before they have an effect. Indeed, when applying extinction, the behavior will often increase before stopping. The therapist who "felt too tired" to block the client from focusing on the past had experienced such a phenomenon previously with the client, but she had not recognized the phenomenon as a behavioral burst and consequently abandoned extinction as a solution. Finally, therapists sometimes apply a solution that stops clients' TIBs in the short term but reinforces the behaviors in the long term. For example, one therapist reported that a client's repeated dissociation during BCAs prevented them from ever completing a BCA. The therapist reported using several grounding techniques that effectively stopped the dissociation, doing a brief BCA on the dissociation that revealed that the client experienced the BCA as "very stressful," and then moving to another topic that the client found less stressful. The team proposed two hypotheses about the repeated dissociation, namely, that the therapist had not taught the client any solutions for "stress" other than stimulus control and that the therapist might have reinforced the dissociation by removing the stimulus of a BCA as a consequence of dissociating. The team then role-played with the therapist how to return to the original BCA after helping the client learn more effective ways to manage the "stress."

CHAPTER 4

SOLUTION ANALYSIS

$\mathbf{D}$BT therapists conduct solution analyses to identify and implement the most effective CBT procedures to change the controlling variables identified through the BCA. The aim in DBT is not just to stop the target behavior and leave the client suffering, but to resolve the issues that contribute to the behavior and relieve the client's suffering as well. This chapter focuses on the general components of solution analyses and common problems in conducting them. Subsequent chapters focus on the application of specific CBT procedures.

SOLUTION ANALYSIS: GENERAL GUIDELINES

Conceptualization and Strategies

Include All Components of a Solution Analysis

Generally, therapists divide a solution analysis into three basic components: the generation, the evaluation, and the implementation of solutions. After selecting a specific link from the chain analysis, the therapist and client generate solutions for that link. The therapist and client may generate as many solutions as possible before evaluating them or evaluate the solutions as they arise. The procedure used will depend on whether interweaving evaluation disrupts solution generation or makes it more efficient. Following the evaluation, the solution is often implemented during the session, although trying the solution first can sometimes provide the best opportunity for evaluation. After the therapist and client have completed the analysis for one link in the chain, they then proceed to select another link. The degree of generation, evaluation, and implementation for each link will vary, but all components should be included in the analysis as a whole. While utilizing the components of solution analyses as therapeutic strategies to treat a specific target, therapists also teach clients how to use these therapeutic strategies as skills to solve other problems themselves and thus reduce the need for prolonged psychotherapy.

Select a Controlling Variable to Resolve

To begin the solution analysis, the therapist and client select a link identified as a controlling variable in the BCA. Factors that influence the selection include how strongly the link appears to control the target behavior, the link's frequency in BCAs, the ease of treating the link, the link's connection to the client's goals, and the client's willingness to address that link (see Table 4.1). For example, a BCA from Anna (the depressed client from Chapter 1 with serotonin problems) identified biochemical changes, depressed mood, social withdrawal, self-invalidation, familial invalidation, shame, the availability of medication for an overdose, and inpatient staff validation all as contributors to her suicide attempt. The therapist wanted to focus first on removing access to sufficient medication for an overdose because this seemed the most critical controlling variable, but Anna adamantly refused to address this because having the medication "made her feel safe." Weighing the relative dangers of letting Anna keep lethal means versus losing Anna's in-session collaboration, the therapist agreed to focus on solving other links first, but added that if Anna persisted in misusing the medication (which she did), they would have to treat access to medication as well (which they did). The therapist then proceeded to the shame link, as the behavioral analysis suggested that the last suicide attempt functioned primarily to reduce shame; the client willingly agreed to focus on this link. They also decided to treat the closely related self-invalidating links because they occurred more frequently than many other links in this chain, as well as in other chains and during therapy sessions. Furthermore, Anna could implement the solutions for self-invalidating thoughts with relative ease. In contrast, Anna's history in other treatments revealed the substantial challenge of changing her depressed mood. Also, the depressed mood was not a good predictor of suicide attempts; though always depressed when attempting suicide, she spent even more time depressed and not attempting suicide. They therefore decided not to work initially on the depressed mood.

The number of links treated in a session will depend on several factors. With newer clients, solution analysis for a single link often

TABLE 4.1. Factors to Consider When Selecting a Link for Solution Analysis

- How strongly the link controls the target behavior.
- The link's frequency across multiple BCAs.
- The ease of treating the link.
- The link's connection to the client's goals.
- The client's willingness to address the link.

progresses slowly, as the therapist must spend more time teaching the client the basics of any new skill or CBT procedure and more time shaping the implementation of the solution. At any point in treatment, TIBs can slow a solution analysis. Some solutions inherently require a substantial time to implement, whereas others require a relatively brief time to implement once the client has learned the basics. For example, formal exposure might require a significant portion of the session, or even its own session. In contrast, changing body posture to change an in-session emotion requires very little time. Breathing exercises and progressive relaxation require only a few minutes. Once learned, mindfulness of judgments, interpretations, and other cognitions require only a minute or two, allowing therapists enough time to ask clients to practice mindfulness multiple times during a session if necessary. Contingency management for in-session TIB may occur almost instantaneously, whereas implementing a contingency management plan for other targets may require substantial planning.

Interweave the Solution Analysis into the BCA

Though the therapist and client can begin the solution analysis after completing the BCA, therapists usually try to interweave the solution and BCAs. Interweaving the two types of analysis has several advantages. It decreases the likelihood that the therapist spends too much time analyzing the causes of the target behavior and consequently fails to have any time for solutions. Clinical experience suggests that it also tends to help the client more quickly begin to identify the link as problematic. Finally, it seems to create a more automatic association between the problematic link and its possible solutions. To decide when to interweave solutions, therapists generally apply the same principles that they use to determine when to treat a controlling variable at all, as described above. In addition, therapists immediately treat variables in the BCA when those variables arise in session during the analysis itself. For example, many clients relate a judgmental thought that occurred during a chain but describe it as a fact rather than as a judgmental thought. In such cases, therapists would weave in practice of noticing judgments, both to change the link in the chain and to block in-session rehearsal and possibly reinforcement of judgmental thinking.

Weave Orienting Strategies into the Solution Analysis

Therapists also interweave solution analyses with orienting strategies (Linehan, 1993a) whenever a solution involves learning about a new skill or a new CBT technique. In the context of the solution analysis, these strategies aim to enhance effective collaboration by teaching clients about the essential elements of any novel solution. Orienting strategies include clarifying the function of the solution, providing relevant theoretical information, specifying the required steps or tasks and highlighting possible temporary side effects. Therapists often use different orienting strategies for different components of the solution analysis. For example, in the case of exposure, a therapist might only orient the client to the function of exposure during solution generation and then review the course of the procedure during solution evaluation. Finally, in preparation for solution implementation, the therapist would clarify the steps or tasks of exposure and alert the client to the possibility of the emotion intensifying before it subsides.

Offer Clients Choices during the Solution Analysis

To enhance collaboration, therapists allow the client as much decision-making control as possible during the solution analysis. A recent review of the empirical literature (Leotti, Iyengar, & Ochsner, 2010) not only validates the "common knowledge" that humans prefer to perceive themselves as in control of a situation, but also presents evidence of an adaptive biological basis for valuing control and having choices. Other recent research (Leotti & Delgado, 2011) has revealed that simply anticipating an opportunity to have a choice increases the activity in areas of the brain associated with reward processing. In DBT, therapists offer clients the opportunity to select the controlling variable for analysis whenever possible. They also usually first ask clients to generate solutions before generating any themselves and allow clients to choose which solutions to implement. Of course, not doing a solution analysis at all is not an option on the menu.

An Illustration: Solution Analysis for Rita

Rita's solution analysis for the target of threatening, in Box 4.1, illustrates a number of these principles. Even before beginning the BCA, the
therapist thought of repair as a contingency management solution for the
threatening behavior, but she also thought that Rita would remain more
collaborative if they first addressed the variables related to the function of the threatening. They started the BCA with a brief summary of
the vulnerabilities and then proceeded through the details of the chain.
When Rita rated anxiety at "3 out of 5," her therapist replied with "This
sounds important. I have a couple of solutions, but they're a bit complex.
Shall we continue with the chain now and watch for simpler solutions
and then return to the anxiety?" Rita readily agreed.

At the first assumption ("He thinks I'm getting worse, that I don't
deserve to be here"), the therapist highlighted it and suggested practicing
mindfulness, as she thought that this skill needed substantial strengthening and that they could practice it quickly. Rita objected, declaring,
"Everything is about skills. I've had enough of skills." The therapist
responded by saying, "Well, we can troubleshoot 'having enough,' or we
can do cognitive restructuring, or we can return to the anxiety and do
something called 'exposure,' which is difficult but very effective." Rita
chose cognitive restructuring and successfully implemented examining
the evidence, which the therapist reinforced with her knowledge of the
psychiatrist's intentions. For the first thought about others not understanding, Rita initially chose examining the evidence again, but when
the implementation seemed more complex than expected, the therapist
offered the choice of generating alternative interpretations instead or
proceeding to the next link. Rita chose to proceed with the BCA.

The therapist had to inhibit her own urge to plunge in with the
emotion regulation skill of "opposite action" when Rita identified anger
as a link. In an earlier, similar analysis, the therapist had generated a
number of solutions for anger and its related links, but later learned
that the anger had occurred as a secondary emotion that functioned
to distract Rita from anxiety. Treating the anger rather than the anxiety had proven an inefficient use of time. The therapist thought that
anger served the same function in this chain and so continued the BCA
without generating more solutions until the target behavior. She again
considered repair as a contingency management strategy, but decided to
postpone this solution. When the therapist learned that the psychiatrist's
response dramatically decreased Rita's anxiety, she thought about trying
to implement extinction, but quickly decided that this solution would

Box 4.1. Solution Analysis for Rita's Threatening	
Links	**Generated solutions**
Psychiatrist says, "I notice that you have self-harmed three times recently on the unit. I'm wondering how you feel things are going here?"	
Anxiety (3/5).	**Exposure.**
Urge to leave (3/5).	
Thinks, "He thinks I'm getting worse, that I don't deserve to be here."	Mindfulness, **examining the evidence**.
Anxiety increases (5/5).	**Exposure.**
Thinks, "I'm working as hard as I can."	
Thinks, "They don't understand how hard I'm working."	**Examining the evidence**, generating alternative interpretations.
Thinks, "People never understand me."	**Dialectical thinking.**
Thinks, "My team should understand me."	
Anger (3/5).	
Says, "I'm working as hard as I can, but nobody understands me. Everyone just keeps pushing and pushing."	"DEAR MAN GIVE FAST" skills.
Anger (4/5).	
Psychiatrist says, "I'm sure people do realize that it's difficult."	
Anger (5/5).	
Says, "No they don't. My therapist just keeps telling me to stop harming and to use skills, skills, skills. What the f**k does she know?"	"DEAR MAN GIVE FAST" skills.
Says, "I'm going to complain about her bullying me. You all bully me. I'll complain to the hospital managers about the lot of you."	**Repair, "DEAR MAN GIVE FAST"** skills.
Anxiety decreases (4/5).	
Psychiatrist says, "This is obviously all a bit difficult for you today. Maybe we should end now," and then ends the meeting.	Extinguish threatening by no longer ending the meeting (and related anxiety) as a consequence of threatening.
Anxiety decreases (2/5).	
Nurse offers her an as-needed medication and a warm drink.	

(continued)

Box 4.1. (*continued*)

Nurse tells her that the psychiatrist is "very concerned" about her and asks if she understands the complaints procedure.	Extinguish threatening by no longer responding to it with validation that reduces anxiety or anger.
Thinks, "They understand how difficult it is for me now."	
Anxiety decreases (0/5).	
Anger decreases (0/5).	

Note. **Bold font = solutions implemented;** standard font = solutions generated only.

require a significant investment for an uncertain return. She had the same thoughts about the nurse's intervention.

With a clearer understanding of the function of Rita's behavior at this point, the therapist offered Rita help to address her anxiety or to use interpersonal effectiveness skills to achieve her goal of obtaining validation from the psychiatrist about her distress and her difficulties. Rita still disliked the idea of skills, though connecting them to her goals did interest her. She decided to address the original anxiety, focusing particularly on reducing the unwarranted portion of her anxiety. The therapist began by saying, "I would have suggested acting opposite, but if you don't want more skills, we can apply a procedure called exposure instead," and she then oriented Rita to the procedure. When Rita rejected exposure because it would initially increase her anxiety, her therapist connected the solution to Rita's long-term goals and guided her through an objective evaluation of the solution. With Rita's agreement, they implemented the solution. Finally, the therapist returned to the contingency of a repair and helped Rita to apply her interpersonal skills to write an apology.

Common Problems with Solution Analysis in General

As with conducting BCAs, conceptual and strategic problems commonly occur when therapists analyze solutions. Although many of these problems relate to a specific component of solution analyses, some problems relate to solution analyses more generally. These problems include failing to conduct a solution analysis, conducting an overgeneralized analysis, and focusing the solution analysis on a less causal portion of the BCA. They also include not interweaving the solution analysis with the BCA, not providing sufficient orientation to solutions, and not connecting the analysis to the client's goals.

Failing to Conduct a Solution Analysis

The biggest problem, particularly common among novice therapists, is failing to include any solution analysis at all. This problem occurs for several reasons. Therapists with a background in insight therapies may become absorbed in the BCA instead of pursuing the solution analysis. DBT, however, does not propose that insight functions as the primary mechanism of change. Some therapists aim to complete a perfect chain analysis or find *the* key controlling variable (both impossible) before pursing the solution analysis. Successful problem solving in DBT requires that the therapist remember that the chain analysis serves the solution analysis, and not the other way around. If the therapist knows the function of the behavior and the link most closely related to the function, the therapist has enough links to begin a solution analysis. Sometimes, time seems simply to slip away. If this problem occurs regularly, external prompts can help. For example, therapists might set an alarm to buzz midway through the session as a prompt to do at least some solution analysis before returning to the chain analysis. Therapists with no or little CBT experience often prolong the chain analysis to avoid the solution analysis because they do not know which solutions to generate or how to implement the solutions. Similarly, these therapists often fear how the clients will react to the solution analysis. The consultation team can help significantly with this problem. For example, one therapist admitted to her team that she avoided the solution analysis because she often had the experience of "running out" of solutions. To address this issue, the team first reviewed the principles of solution generation (covered later in this chapter) and provided the therapist with several models of comprehensive solution analyses. They also assigned relevant homework, namely, that the therapist practice generating as many solutions as possible for a set of BCAs that they had given her. Next, they shaped her new solution generation and continued with similar assignments until the therapist no longer struggled to generate solutions during sessions.

Generating Solutions Only at a General Level

Some therapists produce only a general set of solutions, a set that focuses on the BCA as a whole rather than on specific links. In these circumstances, therapists have usually completed the BCA and then begun the "solution analysis" with a global question such as "What could you have done differently?" rather than questions such as "Which link would be the most useful to work on first?" or suggesting a link to begin the analysis. These global sets of solutions fail to benefit from the analytical aspect of problem solving, which identifies particular variables as having more of a controlling or mediating impact. The global approach therefore risks wasting time on less important links. General solution generation also increases the likelihood of producing solutions that do not fit links in the chain. For example, one therapist had correctly identified all of the cognitive links during the BCA, but rather than analyze appropriate solutions, she globally suggested mindfulness and cognitive restructuring for all of the cognitions. In reviewing her solution analysis, the consultation team highlighted several cognitions, particularly judgmental thoughts, for which DBT would not suggest cognitive restructuring. Another therapist recommended mindfulness and acting opposite as global solutions for the client's emotions and failed to evaluate the appropriateness of these solutions for each emotional link. The consultation team, however, highlighted that the circumstances warranted one of the emotional responses and that stimulus control would likely prove more effective, as well as more validating to the client.

Focusing Analysis on Distal Variables

Other therapists tend to focus their solution analysis on a behavioral chain's more distal variables that have a relatively weak causal connection to the target behavior. This problem often occurs when therapists overly emphasize the vulnerability factors during the BCA, as discussed in Chapter 3. The problem can also occur when therapists complete the BCA and then arbitrarily start the solution analysis with the beginning of the chain rather than first analyzing which variables have the strongest causal relationship to the target behavior. Consultation teams can help to address these two reasons by reviewing solution analyses and reminding therapists to start these analyses with the links that have the strongest causal relationship to the target. Trying to interweave solutions can also lead to this problem if the therapist begins the BCA with the prompting event and works forward chronologically. In this case, the problem usually does not result from a conceptual error but from simply not having enough time to complete the BCA while interweaving solutions from beginning to end. Therapists can reduce the likelihood of this problem occurring by starting the BCA closer to the target behavior and then working back toward the prompting event. Alternatively, the therapist could continue to work forward with the BCA, but become more selective about when to interweave solutions. This often happens naturally, as multiple analyses with a client allows the therapist to recognize when interweaving solutions will prove most efficient.

Not Interweaving Solutions into the BCA

Many therapists struggle to interweave the solution analysis with the BCA. Novice therapists particularly experience the interweaving of the two tasks as overwhelming. Though the literature on learning new skills would validate any decision to separate the two analytical tasks at first, therapists need not wait until they have mastered each task before beginning to combine them. Therapists often benefit from initially trying to interweave only a few types of solutions, such as those solutions that they know best. Some therapists decide to focus first on solutions that seem to have the most immediate impact on clients or that they can implement most easily or quickly. For example, regulating breathing and changing body posture has an immediate impact on many clients, and most therapists elicit these skills from clients with relative speed and ease. Many therapists focus initially on weaving in mindfulness because, with a little more practice, it too can require little time to implement but have an immediate impact.

Failing to Orient Clients to Solutions

Some problems that occur during solution analyses result from not including sufficient orientation to the solutions. For example, many therapists have assumed that their clients have had sufficient orientation to mindfulness because their clients attended the relevant skills training groups. During solution evaluation, however, many clients reject mindfulness as a solution due to a problem with orientation to the skill. Some clients have experienced mindfulness as ineffective because they have misunderstood the function of mindfulness and expect it to function as an emotion regulation skill or a "thought-stopping" technique, and thus they reject the skill when it does not meet their inaccurate expectations. Other clients have believed that they cannot succeed at mindfulness because they have noticed becoming distracted when trying mindfulness, and they have assumed that this indicates failure rather than realizing that this indicates success at noticing distraction. During solution implementation to exposure, therapists sometimes fail to orient to, and consequently prepare for, the likelihood that the intensity of clients' emotions temporarily will increase further. This failure of orientation decreases the likelihood that clients will tolerate the increased emotional intensity. If therapists omit orientation only occasionally, they can correct the omission as it occurs. If the problem occurs regularly, however, therapists may benefit from reviewing the orientation points for each type of solution and role-playing orientation with the consultation team.

Failing to Link Solutions to Client Goals

Finally, conflict between a therapist and client frequently arises if the therapist pursues some aspect of the solution analysis that distresses the client without sufficiently establishing a connection between that aspect of the analysis and the client's goals. For example, early in treatment with Amanda, an outpatient, her therapist tried to focus the solution analysis on Amanda's judgmental thoughts. Amanda, however, refused to generate any solutions because she viewed these thoughts as a fundamental part of her personality that she did not want to change. The therapist then realized that he had failed to connect changing the judgmental thoughts with either Amanda's immediate goal of reducing her self-harm urges (the target of the analysis) or her longer-term goal of establishing lasting relationships. After he highlighted how the judgmental thoughts related to these goals, Amanda's willingness to address the judgmental thoughts notably increased. To further enhance Amanda's willingness to treat the judgmental thoughts, the therapist then attended to her thoughts about changing her personality.

SOLUTION GENERATION

Conceptualization and Strategies

Having selected a controlling variable for treatment, the therapist and client begin the process of generating solutions. The therapist and client generate as many solutions as possible from the full range of CBT procedures that match the controlling variables and the context in which they occur. Within the analysis as a whole and frequently for a single link, therapists attend to balancing acceptance and change solutions. Often therapists must treat clients' difficulties with solution generation itself. Key points in solution generation are listed in Table 4.2.

Match the Solution to the Type of Link and the Context

Matching controlling variables with their respective solutions first assumes, of course, that the therapist and client have correctly differentiated and labeled affect, cognitions, and impulses. DBT solution generation also requires therapists to apply behavioral theory to determine which type of CBT procedure or other solution best matches the selected controlling variable. The standard CBT procedures used in DBT include skills training, stimulus control, exposure, cognitive restructuring, and contingency management. If the selected link in the chain occurs because

TABLE 4.2. Key Points in Solution Generation

- Match solutions to links.
  - Match type of CBT procedure(s) to type of link.
  - Match solution to intensity of link.
  - Match solution to environmental context for use.
- Generate specific, rather than general, skills and other CBT procedures.
- Generate multiple solutions for a single link when possible.
- Balance change and acceptance solutions within an analysis.
- Include a range of skills and other CBT procedures across solution analyses.

the client lacks the skills to respond more effectively, the therapist teaches the required skills. If the client has the required skills but does not use them because of motivational issues, the therapist considers other CBT solutions. For example, when external or internal stimuli motivate problematic behavior or inhibit skillful behavior, the therapist could suggest stimulus control. If a stimulus elicits an unwarranted emotion that then motivates a target behavior or inhibits skills use, the therapist could apply exposure procedures. For faulty cognitions, the therapist could use cognitive modification. If the environment has either punished or not reinforced skillful behavior or has reinforced problematic behavior, then the therapist could consider contingency management procedures.

After choosing the general type of CBT procedure, therapists and clients select more specific techniques within the general procedure. For example, Rita's solution analysis in Box 4.1 specifies examining evidence rather than the broad category of cognitive restructuring, "DEAR MAN GIVE FAST" skills rather than interpersonal effectiveness skills, and extinction rather than contingency management (see Linehan, 2014, for details of the acronym). This refinement often continues throughout the analysis. Selecting the best matching solutions requires that the therapist have a thorough understanding of the function of each specific CBT procedure, including each skill.

A successful analysis also requires therapists to generate solutions appropriate to the contexts in which clients will apply the solutions. Contextual factors include internal and external factors. For example, a client might need to use different interpersonal skills depending on whether he or she is speaking with family members, a physician, or a drug dealer. Mindfulness and emotion regulation techniques that work at home may not work while driving or dining in a restaurant. Clients usually need different emotion regulation skills when they have high emotional intensity compared with low intensity. Though selecting from such a relatively broad spectrum of procedures to find the best match for the diverse causes and contexts of target behaviors makes the therapy more difficult to learn, considering multiple problem-solving options is consistent with research indicating that individuals who flexibly use different types of solutions in different situations both cope better in specific stressful situations and have better general mental health (see Kashdan & Rottenberg, 2010, for a review).

Combine Different Solutions for the Same Link

Many links warrant a combination of different types of solutions. For example, when Anna and her therapist addressed the shame elicited by her family's criticism, they decided that the facts did not justify shame because Anna had not done anything "wrong." For this unjustified shame, they generated the skill of acting opposite and exposure as solutions. When they generated solutions for Anna's self-invalidating thoughts, they included mindfulness skills (e.g., mindfully labeling the thought, describing the facts) and cognitive restructuring (e.g, examining evidence for the thoughts, increasing validating thoughts). Of course, the delineation between what constitutes a skill versus another CBT procedure differs according to theoretical perspective. For example, from a skills training perspective, much of cognitive restructuring involves teaching clients cognitive skills, whereas a cognitive therapist might consider the mindfulness skills as a particular type of cognitive modification. The emotion regulation skill of "acting opposite" closely resembles key elements of exposure. DBT therapists do not try to resolve these theoretical debates and instead concern themselves with how each theory and its techniques can help to solve part of the clinical puzzle.

Balance Acceptance and Change Solutions

When conducting the solution analysis, therapists attempt to generate a dialectical set of solutions that balance acceptance and change. The combination of mindfulness as an acceptance skill and cognitive restructuring as a change procedure for Anna's self-invalidating thoughts exemplifies such a dialectical balance. Emma, an inpatient, assumed that the other female patients in her skills training group disliked her because they knew about her extramarital affairs. The thought elicited shame during the group, which then caused the patient to miss group. Like

Anna's therapist, Emma's therapist suggested the dialectical pairing of cognitive restructuring and mindfulness for the problematic cognition. The cognitive restructuring included examining the evidence for Emma's assumption and challenging her catastrophic thinking. Mindfulness included identifying the thought as a thought and instead focusing on the task at hand (i.e., either preparing for, going to, or participating in group). Implementation of these solutions revealed that examining the evidence worked well when Emma had no evidence (most clients did not dislike her), but that the mindfulness worked better when she did have evidence. Challenging the catastrophic thinking did not help either way. Emma also experienced intense guilt about her affairs because of the impact that they had on her husband. She had repeatedly attempted suicide to stop the guilt.

The emphasis on considering both acceptance and change-based solutions may prove particularly important when treating emotional links. Research (Bonanno, Papa, Lalande, Westphal, & Coifman, 2004; Westphal, Seivert, & Bonanno, 2010) has indicated that individuals who flexibly choose between enhancing versus suppressing emotional expression based on the situation have better long-term adjustment. In contrast to Anna's unjustified shame, the facts did justify a substantial portion of Emma's guilt, as her behavior had harmed her husband psychologically and professionally. For the warranted guilt, Emma and her therapist generated solutions to increase the acceptance of the emotion (e.g., mindfully allowing the emotion, radically and willingly accepting it as a consequence of her past behaviors) and to repair the damage to her husband (e.g., becoming more validating toward him, helping him with his work during home visits). Emma also experienced guilt about her husband in situations that did not warrant it. During a home visit, for example, Emma had experienced justified guilt earlier in the evening, but later at night she remained awake staring at her peacefully sleeping husband and ruminating on the impact of her affairs until she felt so guilty that she harmed herself. As the cue (a peacefully sleeping husband) did not justify the emotional response, Emma and her therapist emphasized solutions designed to change the emotion. For the guilt at this point in the chain, they combined stimulus control and exposure. Stimulus control (i.e., shifting the client's attention away from her husband) provided a short-term solution to prevent self-harm, but it did not change the classically conditioned relationship between the husband's presence and guilt. Exposure did change the conditioned relationship, but it required a longer time to implement.

Treat Clients' Solution-Generation Difficulties

Many clients with BPD struggle with generating solutions. As a result of growing up in invalidating environments, some clients never received adequate modeling of how to generate solutions. Other clients have acquired the basics of solution generation but the behavior remains weak or inhibited because in the past their solutions have failed or have been punished by others. For example, when Joanne, an unemployed client who had just turned 20, suggested higher education as a way to improve her quality of life, her uneducated parents responded by asking "Who do you think you are? Do you think that you are better than us?" Thus, clients' difficulties with solution generation can result from either skills deficits or motivational issues. Clients who lack the relevant skills may benefit from some basic teaching on how to generate solutions (e.g., learning where to look for ideas). Therapists address motivational issues with the corresponding strategies. For example, the client described above inhibited solution generation in the session because she feared that her therapist would invalidate her as well. Because the fear was unwarranted in the context of therapy (i.e., the therapist would not invalidate her), the therapist used exposure, asking the client to continue generating solutions, including unrealistic ones, until the fear subsided. To shape solution generation more generally, therapists reinforce any reasonable attempt by clients to generate solutions and encourage clients to generate as many solutions as possible before evaluating them.

Two Illustrations: Solution Analyses for Jane and Susan

Jane's case exemplifies several principles of solution generation. Box 4.2 illustrates a summary of Jane's solutions generated across multiple BCAs of the target behavior. Jane and her therapist generated specific solutions (e.g., be nonjudgmental, opposite action, examining evidence), indicated by boldface, during the course of the BCA summarized in Box 4.2. During subsequent, but similar BCAs of vomiting, Jane and her therapist generated the solutions in regular text. Compared with Rita, Jane had a longer session and she had learned (but not generalized) a number of solutions through previously targeting suicidal behaviors. Consequently, Jane and her therapist had more time to generate more solutions during her initial solution analysis for vomiting, although they did not implement all of the solutions during the session. Although the initial solution analysis did not contain the full range of CBT interventions (it lacked exposure), the summary of all solution analyses for vomiting did include the full range. During the initial analysis, Jane and her therapist did

---

Box 4.2. Solution Analysis for Jane's Vomiting

Links	Generated solutions
Poor sleep.	
Argument with mother.	Many interpersonal effectiveness skills.
Rumination.	Mindfulness of present moment.
Guilt.	Repair.
Views television program about dieting.	**Remove stimulus.**
Anxiety (2/5).	
Scans body.	Urge surfing.
Views advertisement on television.	
Urge to check whether jeans fit.	**Urge surfing.**
Tries on jeans.	Remove stimulus.
Feel and sight of jeans not fitting.	
Fear (3/5).	Exposure, opposite action.
Feels queasy.	
Thinks, "It's no good; I'll always be fat."	**Mindfulness,** examining the evidence.
Looks at herself in the mirror, scanning for evidence of "fat places."	Urge surfing, reorient attention.
Repeatedly labels "fat" areas.	Be nonjudgmental.
Fear increases (4/5).	**TIP skills for physiology,** opposite action.
Thinks, "I'm always going to be fat."	**Mindfulness,** examining the evidence.
Thinks, "I have no control."	**Build mastery,** examining the evidence, dialectical thinking.
Shame (3/5).	
Thinks, "Mom's right. I'm selfish, hopeless, and too focused on myself."	Be nonjudgmental.
Guilt (3/5).	**Repair,** radical acceptance.
Sits on bed with head in her hands.	**Opposite action.**
Notices her stomach "spilling out" of the jeans.	
Thinks, "See that just proves I'm out of control. Look at me. Mom was right."	Mindfulness, examining the evidence.
Shame increases (4/5).	**Opposite action.**
"Replays" the previous days argument with her mother.	**Focus on present task of implementing repair.**
Thinks, "How can I be so critical of Mom? She just tries to help me."	

(continued)

Box 4.2. (*continued*)

Guilt (4/5).	Repair, opposite action.
Thinks, "I owe her everything."	Dialectical thinking.
Thinks, "Just think of all the trouble I've caused."	**Focus on present task of implementing repair,** radical acceptance.
Ruminates about past events.	**Focus on present.**
Thinks, "John [her brother] left because of me. He blames me for mom being so upset."	Radical acceptance, focus on present moment.
Guilt increases (5/5).	**TIP skills, opposite action.**
Thinks, "I have an unpayable debt to Mom. There's nothing I can do."	Dialectical thinking.
Thinks, "I should be punished for what I've done."	Be nonjudgmental.
Urge to vomit (4/5).	**Urge surfing, phone therapist,** review negative consequences.
Goes to the bathroom to vomit.	**Walk away from bathroom.**
Vomits spontaneously at the sight of the toilet.	
Fear decreases (3/5).	
Queasiness decreases.	
Thinks, "Now I'm in control."	**Extinguish overdosing by restructuring belief about being in control that subsequently decreases shame.**
Shame decreases (3/5).	
Thinks, "It's not enough."	
Puts fingers down her throat and vomits twice.	Opposite action.
Feels tired.	
Fear decreases (1/5), shame decreases (1/5).	
Thinks, "This is the punishment I deserve."	**Extinguish overdosing by restructuring belief that punishment has occurred and justifies decreased guilt.**
Guilt decreases (1/5).	
Returns to the bedroom and goes to sleep.	

Note. **Bold font = specific solutions generated in initial analysis;** standard font = solutions generated in subsequent analyses of similar episodes.

succeed, however, in producing a dialectical set of solutions, including radical acceptance and mindfulness-based solutions on the acceptance side and emotion regulation-based solutions, challenging cognitions, and extinction on the other.

The selection of links for solution generation, and the generated solutions, depended on many of the factors described in the introduction to solution analysis. In the initial analysis, Jane and her therapist focused on links in the chain rather than vulnerability factors, as the former had a clearer causal relationship to the vomiting. The therapist further focused her initial solution generation on solutions that had a likelihood of being relatively easy or effective for Jane. Both the client's existing capabilities and the time required for implementation affected the therapist's assessment of ease. Jane often experienced mindfulness as easier than cognitive restructuring, so her therapist suggested mindfulness more in the initial analysis. Because exposure would have required more time than changing physiology and opposite action, the therapist waited until subsequent analyses to suggest exposure. Jane's history of success with solutions, both prior to and during the session, and the intensity of her emotions and urges in the BCA influenced the therapist's assessment of probable effectiveness. Previous BCAs of other targets had revealed that Jane struggled to use mindfulness more whenever she thought "Mom's right," so neither Jane nor her therapist suggested mindfulness for such links in the initial analysis. Within the session itself, the therapist suggested urge surfing for the urge to try on the jeans, but Jane anticipated that she would struggle to implement this solution, so the therapist did not suggest it for the scanning urge. They did return to the solution, however, for the vomiting urges because these urges so strongly controlled the target behavior that the therapist thought that they needed a solution for that link. Finally, the intensity of Jane's emotions and urges influenced the solutions generated for a particular link. In general, the therapist emphasized solutions requiring cognitive capacity (e.g., mindfulness, radical acceptance) when the emotions remained lower and emphasized changing physiological arousal more when the emotions had escalated. She did not generate dialectical thinking as a solution in the initial analysis because the links for which it could have proved helpful all occurred during times of high emotional intensity when Jane would have had great difficulty implementing the solution.

Susan's case also demonstrates solution-generation principles. Box 4.3 shows a summary of the solutions generated across multiple BCAs of suicidal behaviors involving infidelity. Susan had familiarity with some of the solutions from previous BCAs of suicidal behaviors prompted by other events. She and her therapist generated the solutions in boldface during the initial solution analysis for the overdose involving infidelity and the other solutions during subsequent, but similar BCAs. The solutions in bold from the initial analysis illustrate how a single solution analysis can contain a range of solutions; Susan's analysis includes all types of CBT solutions except exposure. Furthermore, the analysis refines the solutions beyond their broad CBT category. For example, Susan's analysis specifies being nonjudgmental and urge surfing rather than mindfulness, radical acceptance and distraction rather than distress tolerance, and extinction rather than contingency management. The original solutions also demonstrate a dialectical balance that includes mindfulness and distress-tolerance skills on the acceptance side and emotion regulation skills, cognitive restructuring, and contingency management on the change side. During the initial analysis, Susan and her therapist did not generate solutions for the vulnerability factors, except for the link of agreeing to take the man home, which was a key controlling variable in the BCA. Like Jane's therapist, Susan's therapist generally emphasized fewer cognitive solutions at points of higher emotional intensity, but she made an exception for the "don't deserve to live" link because the urge to overdose followed immediately. Though she knew that the thought could have resulted from the guilt or fear with no causal relationship to the urge, she hypothesized that such a causal relationship had existed.

Common Problems in Solution Generation

Conceptual Errors

One set of common problems with solution analyses results from conceptual errors regarding solution generation. These errors can result in solutions that do not match the causal variables, oversimplify the complexity of the problem, or have insufficient specificity. As a group, these errors decrease the likelihood that clients will have sufficient solutions to achieve their goals, that their solutions will prove rewarding, and that they will persist with solution implementation. Reviews of solution analyses often provide an efficient means for consultation teams to identify and subsequently treat such errors.

MISMATCHING CONTROLLING VARIABLES, SOLUTIONS, AND CONTEXTS

A mismatch between a controlling variable and the solutions generated for it can occur if the therapist mislabels the controlling variable, does not attend to the emotional intensity or environmental context of the

---

Box 4.3. Solution Analysis for Susan's Overdose

Links	Generated solutions
Argument with her boyfriend.	Many interpersonal effectiveness skills.
Thinks relationship will end.	Mindfulness, examining the evidence.
Anxiety.	
Disagreement with individual therapist.	
Anger.	
Drinking.	
Agrees to take a male stranger home.	**Review negative consequences, say "No," stimulus control.**
Happy.	
Has sex with man at home.	Say "No."
Thinks, "I shouldn't have sex with someone else."	Letting go, radical acceptance.
Guilt (4/5).	**TIP skills to change physiology, reorient attention/distraction, repair.**
Urge to self-harm (3/5).	Urge surfing.
Thinks, "I'll feel better if I harm."	Review negative consequences.
Curls up in bed.	
Hears man move.	**Remove stimulus with "DEAR MAN" skills.**
Thinks, "I'm a cheat."	Radical acceptance.
Guilt increases (5/5), shame (5/5).	**TIP skills to change physiology, reorient attention/distraction, opposite action.**
Thinks, "I don't deserve him anyway."	Be nonjudgmental.
Thinks, "I don't even deserve to live."	**Be nonjudgmental.**
Urge to self-harm increases (4/5).	Review negative consequences.
Goes to the bathroom to overdose.	
Takes 30 antidepressant pills.	**Keep minimal pills** and list of negative consequences with pill bottle.
Guilt decreases (3/5), shame decreases (3/5).	
Man enters bathroom, appraises situation, calls paramedics, and leaves.	
Sensation of sickness and wooziness.	*(continued)*

Box 4.3. (*continued*)

Paramedics arrive, administer treatment, and take her to the hospital.	
Assessed and admitted to the psychiatric ward.	
Thinks, "I deserve being stuck here as a punishment."	**Extinguish overdosing by restructuring belief that punishment has occurred and justifies decreased guilt.**
Guilt decreases (2/5).	
Boyfriend visits and tells her that he's learned the "whole story," but forgives her because she "must have been really sorry" if she "tried to kill" herself.	Extinguish overdosing by no longer responding to it with forgiveness that reduces guilt or shame or creates a sense of connection.
Guilt decreases (1/5), shame decreases (2/5).	
Experiences strong connection to boyfriend.	

Note. **Bold font = specific solutions generated in initial analysis**; standard font = solutions generated in subsequent analyses of similar episodes.

variable, or does not consider the CBT principles of when to use which type of solution. The section above on solution generation highlights the general principles of when to use which solutions. Even if a therapist correctly applies CBT principles to match solutions with controlling variables, however, a mismatch can occur if the therapist tries to generate solutions for a mislabeled controlling variable. For example, if the therapist just labels "feeling abandoned" as an emotion rather than differentiating the thought from the emotion, the therapist might fail to consider cognitive restructuring. The therapist might also generate emotion-based solutions that will not work because thoughts of abandonment can elicit a variety of emotions, each with its own specific solutions, and the therapist has not identified the specific emotion. Similarly, if a client says "I had an urge to hit him," the therapist might just label this as a thought and suggest only cognitive solutions, not realizing that the client used this statement to communicate an impulse or action urge. As impulses and cognitions arise from different parts of the brain, they often respond better to different solutions. Finally, a therapist might mislabel a valid link as invalid, or vice versa. In Emma's case, her thoughts that the other female patients in her skills training group disliked her because of her extramarital affairs had little to no validity, so cognitive restructuring matched the problem. In another case, however, Jack, a patient in a long-term secure psychiatric unit, believed that all of the unit staff hated him and wanted him off of the unit. The belief frequently appeared as a link leading to suicidal and assaultive urges. Initially, Jack's therapist identified the belief as a cognitive distortion and consequently tried cognitive restructuring. This solution failed, however, as a review of the evidence revealed that about 80% of the staff disliked Jack and wanted him moved off of the unit because of his assaultive, threatening, and otherwise disruptive behaviors on the unit. Thus Jack's beliefs had significant validity. The therapist still wanted to decrease the ruminating because of the link to self-harm, but did not want to invalidate the valid and thus excluded traditional cognitive restructuring. The therapist began by accepting the valid aspects of Jack's thoughts, but then highlighted the ineffective consequences of ruminating, even on valid beliefs. With coaching, Jack learned to describe the thoughts and their consequences more mindfully and to refocus his attention on more effective ways of resolving his conflict with the staff.

Therapists can also generate inappropriate solutions if they fail to attend to the intensity of a controlling variable, particularly emotions. In their work on the tasks of emotion regulation, Gottman and Katz (1990) describe how the intensity of an emotion impacts the ability to accomplish the tasks of emotion regulation. As an emotion escalates, the ability to accomplish tasks with a more cognitive element diminishes. Individuals at the height of an emotion often first need solutions requiring few cognitive demands. For example, when Alexandra's boyfriend made invalidating comments, she always became angry and sometimes became violent. If she experienced moderate anger, she could inhibit any violent urges and reduce her anger by using a variety of stimulus control and emotion regulation skills, including modifying both the salience and the meaning of the stimulus (the invalidating statements), and replacing her own judgmental thoughts with validating thoughts, all of which required a notable amount of thinking. If she experienced extreme anger, however, she had to rely first on skills that directly decreased her physiological arousal (e.g., breathing and relaxation exercises, walking) and skills that removed or distracted her from the stimulus (e.g., leaving the house) to decrease her anger to a moderate level, at which point she could again use a variety of solutions.

Similarly, therapists can generate solutions that conceptually match the controlling variables but mismatch the environmental contexts in which clients will use the solutions. For example, Harmon-Jones and Peterson (2009) reported that students in a supine body position had significantly lower neural responses to negative feedback about themselves and their performance compared with students in an upright position. Suggesting that a client lie down in order to decrease verbally aggressive urges may prove effective at home during a phone call with a family member, but could cause new problems if used at the office while receiving critical feedback from a boss. Many skills that orient clients away from the current context can have negative or even potentially catastrophic consequences in some situations. For example, focusing on breathing effectively reduces emotional arousal, and mindfulness "exercises" (as opposed to being mindful of the current context) effectively reduce judgmental thinking, but practicing these skills in the context of driving could endanger the client and others alike. In some instances, clients may be able to change the context in order to implement the solution (e.g., a driving client could leave the road temporarily), but solutions that work in the current context may prove more effective in the long term.

RESTRICTING THE RANGE OF SOLUTIONS

Just as the biosocial theory proposes that invalidating environments oversimplify the ease of problem solving in general and regulating emotions and impulses in particular, so too can individual therapists oversimplify the solutions required to change target behaviors by restricting the range of solutions. A restricted range of solutions occurs when therapists overrely on one type of solution or generate too few solutions altogether to successfully change the target behavior. Though effective solution generation in DBT does not require every type of CBT solution or a solution for every link in the chain and though some sessions may require more solution implementation and have less time for solution generation, effective *long-term* solution analysis does require that the therapy generate sufficient solutions to address the target behavior's primary function. A single solution seldom proves sufficient in the long term. For example, applying an aversive consequence alone may successfully suppress the behavior in a single context, but such solutions often do not generalize well to other contexts. Removing lethal means from a suicidal client removes the immediate risk, but it does nothing to address the function of the suicidal behavior. If the client does not acquire a solution that addresses the behavior's function as well, the client will likely acquire new lethal means instead.

Overrelying on one type of solution can occur when either the client offers the same default option repeatedly or the therapist suggests a limited set of solutions. Many clients consistently rely on crisis survival skills, particularly at the beginning of treatment. Most clients already know and use some of these skills, and many of these skills have a relative simplicity and immediate impact that makes them appropriate solutions for therapists struggling to coach new clients through crises. Unfortunately, most of the crisis survival skills provide only short-term relief, rather than long-term solutions, and thus, overreliance on these skills will interfere with therapeutic progress. They only help clients to survive crises and not to prevent or resolve crises. As soon as possible, DBT therapists balance these short-term skills with long-term solutions. Clients with BPD also have a tendency to generate solutions that require someone else, such as therapists, social services, or family members, to solve the problem rather than solving it themselves, a pattern that Linehan (1993a) refers to as active passivity. Though such an intervention by others may effectively solve the problem, solutions that rely on external intervention usually do not generalize as well because they require the continued availability and willingness of a third party. For example, Blanche, a psychiatric inpatient on a high-security unit, engaged in several TIBs (e.g., arriving late for therapy, not completing homework, and not implementing skills) that resulted partly from Blanche's "forgetting." Whenever her therapist asked what solutions Blanche could implement to decrease the "forgetting," Blanche always responded that staff could prompt her to engage in the relevant behaviors. Though a prompt from staff would have decreased the immediate instances of the TIB, allowing Blanche to rely on this solution alone would have reinforced her active passivity and would have prolonged her stay on this unit, as less secure units would not have had the resources to provide this level of intervention. In addition to Blanche's solution, her therapist included several solutions that required Blanche doing something different, such as creating visual prompts and alarm reminders. They also arranged some contingency management with the staff such that Blanche received more help from staff when she first actively implemented solutions herself rather than when she just passively waited for others to intervene.

Like clients, therapists sometimes develop an overreliance on certain types of solutions. In some cases, this overreliance occurs because therapists have not yet adequately learned the full range of DBT solutions. For example, a new individual therapist who has no CBT training but has experience coleading a DBT skills group might suggest only skills as solutions and thus treat clients' skills deficits but neglect their motivational issues. A therapist with only cognitive therapy training might rely on cognitive restructuring and minimize skills training or totally neglect exposure or contingency management. Consultation teams can identify and treat such problems by reviewing therapists' solution analyses and then training (e.g., didactic teaching, modeling, role playing) therapists how to apply types of solutions that they have not previously learned. In other cases, overreliance results from therapists becoming especially attached to a type of solution and applying it as a panacea. For example, after learning mindfulness and experiencing the benefits for themselves as well as their clients, many therapists begin to generate mindfulness as a solution for almost every link. Though clients can apply mindfulness to almost any link, mindfulness alone does not change environments, interpersonal relationships, prompting events, and so on. Thus, relying on mindfulness (or any other solution) alone produces a nondialectical solution analysis. Though therapists can monitor and treat such attachments themselves, consultation teams may first notice such patterns and then analyze and treat them. In one case, a brief BCA revealed that the therapist had begun to rely on mindfulness in sessions because she had found mindfulness so helpful in her own life that she assumed that her clients would find it equally helpful. When the team challenged the assumption, the therapist realized that she had underestimated the extent to which she also used a variety of other psychological skills in her own life, but which her clients still lacked. In another case, a consultation team noticed that a therapist had begun to suggest mindfulness as almost the only solution. When simply describing the overreliance as a problem failed to stop the problem, the team conducted a more thorough analysis and discovered that the therapist enjoyed practicing this solution more than any other and that she focused on finding opportunities for it while generating solutions. The therapist agreed to a "ban" on using mindfulness as a solution until she had conducted a certain number of dialectical solution analyses that contained a variety of solutions. This intervention successfully inhibited the therapist from relying on mindfulness and motivated her to become more dialectical.

NOT SPECIFYING SOLUTIONS SUFFICIENTLY

Just as a professional golfer uses a specific club for a specific shot or a carpenter selects certain nails for certain jobs, DBT therapists suggest specific skills or other solutions. Problems often arise if therapists suggest vague solutions, such as an entire module of skills rather than one specific skill from the module. For example, some therapists have simply suggested "emotion regulation skills" as a solution for emotional links in the BCA without proceeding to identify which specific emotion regulation skills will work best. Similarly, some therapists have tended to "challenge" clients' cognitions without clearly helping the client to identify which types of cognitive restructuring to use in which situations. In many cases, this lack of specificity decreases the likelihood that clients will effectively implement the solution during the session and later, either because they are confused by the vagueness of the solution, or because they select a more specific but less effective solution from the larger category. In one case, for example, the therapist simply suggested that the client challenge his cognitions. The client later tried to review the evidence for his beliefs but did not find this helpful because the evidence remained open to interpretation. Meanwhile, the therapist's consultation team had noted the vagueness in the therapist's solution generation and helped him to identify which types of cognitive restructuring to use in which contexts. The therapist then proposed "generating alternative interpretations" to the client, which the client found much more effective. Though in-session solution implementation will usually detect problems resulting from a lack of clarity, specificity during solution generation remains important as sessions seldom have sufficient time to implement all suggested solutions.

Clients' Challenging Responses

NOT TREATING CLIENTS' LACK OF SOLUTION GENERATION

Though therapists seldom have difficulty generating solutions when they conceptually understand the solutions, they frequently encounter challenges from clients when attempting to implement the strategy. They may first encounter challenges when asking clients to generate solutions. The most common problem that arises at this point is that clients respond with "I don't know" or something similar. Though an occasional "I don't know" may result from a client actually not knowing the answer, automatic or constant "I don't knows" usually function as an attempt to avoid solution generation or the subsequent implementation. If the client genuinely does not know, then the therapist should proceed to suggest solutions. Therapists sometimes make a strategic error at this point by pushing too hard or waiting too long for clients to generate solutions because the therapists believe that the solutions must originate from clients' insights. In DBT, however, the solution analysis relies less on clients' insights and more on clients' solution implementation. The source of the solution becomes secondary to having solutions. If the therapist has previously taught the client solutions for a particular link, but the client cannot or does not try to remember them, then the therapist may prompt the client to review the diary card for solutions or develop some other type of prompt. For the client who cannot remember, this solution teaches the client a relevant skill; for the client who does not try to remember, this solution may help to manage any reinforcing contingencies. Similarly, if "I don't know" functions to minimize a client's problem-solving efforts, the therapist might implement contingencies that have the opposite effect. For example, one therapist oriented clients with this function to her policy that failing to generate solutions for an important link indicated to her that the relevant solutions remained weak in their repertoires and that they therefore needed more in-session practice of and homework for these solutions. This policy notably shifted the motivation to generate solutions during sessions for many clients; it also worked well for clients who genuinely did not know the relevant solutions by making those solutions more salient through practice. Frequently, clients do not generate any solutions because they fear that their solutions will seem foolish or that the therapist will judge them. Treatment in such cases can include teaching clients how to return mindfully to solution generation when distracted by solution evaluation; modeling irreverent, potentially foolish solutions (e.g., contacting the therapist with skywriting or singing telegrams if the phone fails); and establishing contingencies that reward clients for simply generating solutions.

MANAGING CLIENTS' PROBLEMATIC SOLUTION GENERATION

When clients do generate solutions, they sometimes suggest rather problematic solutions. They may suggest solutions that will probably not work well for the identified link, such as replacing negative judgments with positive judgments or using crisis survival skills when the situation requires emotion regulation skills. They may also suggest solutions that may cause new problems, such as asking for hospital admission any time they experience suicidal urges. Because therapists want to encourage rather than inhibit client solution generation, they often accept any reasonable option offered by the client during this step and add any more effective solutions themselves, waiting until the next step to evaluate the relative effectiveness of each solution. If a problematic pattern of poor solution generation emerges, however, the therapist may need to shape the behavior sooner rather than later. Occasionally, clients suggest using other target behaviors, such as abusing drugs instead of attempting suicide or using laxatives rather than vomiting. If this behavior appears to function to derail the solution generation, therapists may effectively extinguish the behavior by responding matter-of-factly and continuing with the solution generation. For example, a therapist might respond by saying "Okay, that's one solution. What other solutions have you learned?" Often, however, clients intend nothing more than a bit of humor, in which case a reinforcing response may help the relationship and everyone's mood more than it will interfere with solution generation.

SOLUTION EVALUATION

Conceptualization and Strategies

After generating solutions for an identified controlling variable, therapists and clients proceed to evaluate the solutions for that variable. Although most individuals generally move rapidly between generating and evaluating solutions, problem-solving therapies distinguish between these two behaviors and often treat them as distinct steps to reduce the likelihood of one behavior impeding the other. Unmindfully or impulsively interjecting solution evaluation tends to inhibit solution generation in general and creativity in particular. Not all solutions, however, will prove equally viable. When clients try to implement inappropriate solutions, they fail to solve the current problem and risk having their solution generation and implementation behaviors extinguished or even punished. Thus, therapists teach clients how to evaluate solutions to maximize the likelihood that clients will successfully solve problems. Key components of solution evaluation include reviewing the probable outcomes of a solution to determine the solution's potential efficacy and assessing any factors that might interfere with the solution's implementation. Though discussions may suffice to determine a solution's efficacy or to identify factors that could decrease the effectiveness, an in-session implementation of the solution often allows therapists and clients to more accurately evaluate the solution.

Review the Solution's Probable Consequences

Therapists review the likely proximate and distal consequences of proposed solutions to determine the probability of those solutions successfully treating the relevant controlling variables and helping clients to achieve their goals. The evaluation considers the likelihood of a solution's success based on the conceptual match between the problem and the solution in a given context and on the client's personal experience of using the solution appropriately. For example, cognitive restructuring as a solution conceptually matches an automatic assumption as a problem. Sometimes, however, clients have a history of applying cognitive restructuring correctly, but the assumption persists. In such instances, the evaluation would suggest focusing instead on mindfulness or another solution.

The review emphasizes examining the intermediate and long-term consequences of solutions, partially to correct the tendency of clients to focus on an intervention's immediate impact and neglect the longer-term effects. For example, many clients report that they self-harm because it immediately reduces their negative emotions. In the long term, however, self-harm usually leads to more problems that then elicit more negative emotions. Some clients consider hospitalization the best solution for suicidal urges because hospitalization prevents suicidal behavior for most clients and often provides them with an immediate sense of safety. Unfortunately, they seldom consider whether hospitalization as a response to suicidal urges may actually decrease their safety in the long term because elements of hospitalization have reinforcing consequences for becoming suicidal. Some clients will reject any new skill because they focus on the immediate consequences of learning (e.g., expending effort; experiencing worry, frustration, or disappointment), rather than the intermediate consequences of having learned a new skill (e.g., skillfully solving a problem). When clients compare new solutions with old target behaviors and judge the new solutions as more difficult, less immediate, or less reliable, therapists can still obtain favorable votes for the new solutions by connecting the new solutions to clients' more global, long-term goals.

Therapists also consider the viability of solutions with respect to whether a solution will likely generalize across contexts and time. For example, Blanche's solution of relying on hospital staff to remind her of appointments and homework would not generalize to an environment with fewer staff or less structure. Though not all solutions in the analysis require generalization, at least some of them require this quality. Thus, Blanche's solution analysis included a variety of solutions that she could continue to implement as she progressed to less secure units.

This review of probable consequences offers therapists the best opportunity to shape any questionable solutions generated by clients. It prompts clients to identify the potential problematic consequences before the therapist does so. If therapists need to highlight potential problems with clients' solutions, they balance the critical feedback with validation (of the valid, not the invalid), but avoid treating the client as too fragile to hear the feedback. For example, a therapist might say "Challenging negative judgments with positive judgments might help in this moment, but I'm concerned that this solution keeps you judgmental and leaves you more vulnerable to having other negative judgments. Let's also try mindfully letting go of judgmental thoughts."

Assess Obstacles to a Solution's Implementation

Another component of solution evaluation is the assessment of any factors that will likely interfere with implementing solutions successfully. Clients may lack the skill, the motivation, or practical resources to implement a solution. When the therapist or client has identified an obstacle, they then can either remove or circumvent that obstacle or switch to another solution, based on the difficulty of tackling the obstacle and the viability of other solutions. For example, many clients automatically attend to potential negative outcomes more than potential positive outcomes and anticipate failure. If a client responds with such an automatic cognitive bias to most suggested solutions, then the therapist has little choice but to treat this bias. In contrast, an adult client may not yet have learned sufficient interpersonal skills to decrease the frequent invalidation of a sibling, but may have the capacity to minimize contact with and use mindfulness skills during contact with the sibling. In such a case the therapist and client may decide to forgo developing more advanced interpersonal skills at this time and instead focus on using the other solutions.

Sometimes clients have not yet learned the skills that therapists have suggested, whereas other times clients have partially learned the skills, but misapply them through a lack of either knowledge or practice. In either case, the individual therapist uses skills training to treat the skills deficit. For example, one client experienced problematic levels of conflict with her colleagues. When her therapist suggested using validation to improve her relationships, the client declared that validation would not work. The therapist then suggested that they rehearse validation anyway to better assess exactly why it would not work. This rehearsal immediately revealed that while the client used validating words, she also used what many would label as a "dismissive" tone. The therapist then coached her on how to alter her tone to increase the likelihood of her colleagues responding favorably to her attempts at validation.

Often clients have sufficient skills to use a solution, but motivational issues interfere. Cognitions or emotions may inhibit implementing the solution, or environmental contingencies may not reinforce or may even punish using the solution. Alexandra's case (the client with intense anger and an invalidating boyfriend) illustrates how high emotional arousal creates an obstacle to solutions that require notable cognitive capacity and how therapists might remove this obstacle. Her cognitions also created obstacles themselves, initially leading to a refusal to rehearse the skill at all. When her therapist first suggested that Alexandra use validation as one solution to reduce interpersonal conflict with her boyfriend, Alexandra immediately rejected the solution. A brief analysis of the refusal revealed that Alexandra immediately had the thought "He doesn't deserve validation" when the therapist suggested the solution. The therapist highlighted the judgmental thought and suggested that Alexandra mindfully let go of it and focus on effectiveness, but Alexandra refused to practice these skills. Additional analysis revealed that Alexandra maintained the judgments because they provided her with self-validation. The therapist then encouraged Alexandra to practice other self-validating statements that did not involve judging her boyfriend or being ineffective. After this, Alexandra stopped objecting to validation as a solution.

Sometimes the motivational obstacle originates within the environment rather than within the client. Some environments ignore or even punish solutions that other environments would reward. Many clients have this experience when they use solutions related to assertiveness, even when they apply the solutions with some sophistication. As with other obstacles, the therapist and client can decide to try to remove the obstacle, move around it, or move on to other solutions. For example, Marie had chosen a career option that her talents justified but that her bank balance could not initially finance. The most obvious solution required her to ask her parents for short-term financial support, but the solution evaluation revealed that although her parents had financially supported her treatment since early adolescence, they had also dismissed most of her career goals as "too artsy." Because of the importance of the goal and the limited number of other solutions, however, she decided to try to remove the obstacle of her parents' dismissal. With the therapist's agreement, Marie invited her parents to a therapy session and presented her plan to them. Rather than passively waiting for their dismissal, she actively asked them for their critical feedback and thus partly reduced the aversive quality of their feedback by taking more control of it. She also reduced the extent to which their feedback punished her request by viewing the feedback as patrons considering an investment rather than as parents judging a child. Having neutralized the initial impact of her parents' responses, Marie validated their feedback and addressed the issues that they raised whenever possible. Her parents then agreed to support her financially with certain reasonable conditions. In contrast, Joanne, whose parents ridiculed her higher-education goal, decided to move around the obstacle of her parents' objections by seeking financial and psychological support from other sources.

Emma's case demonstrates several components of solution evaluation in combination. Historically, whenever Emma threatened self-harm or sobbed in front of her husband, she quickly and reliably experienced a reduction in domestic demands and stress, with no immediate sense of guilt. When Emma's therapist suggested using interpersonal skills instead to reduce domestic demands, Emma immediately rejected the solution because she "would feel guilty" using them and they "probably wouldn't work." Emma's therapist then assessed the accuracy of "probably won't work" and discovered that using the skills would probably reduce domestic demands, though perhaps not as quickly or reliably as suicidal threats or sobbing. She also assessed whether using the skills warranted any guilt and determined that it did not on this occasion. Next, Emma's therapist compared the long-term consequences for Emma's marriage of applying assertion skills versus communicating suicidal urges and sobbing and reminded her of her goal of improving her marriage. When Emma refocused her attention on her long-term marital goals, her evaluation of assertion as a solution notably improved. Through a combination of mindfulness, acting opposite to the emotion and cognitive restructuring, Emma and her therapist then tackled her unwarranted guilt as an obstacle to using the skills. Finally, Emma and her therapist role-played the relevant interpersonal skills, so that her therapist could better evaluate whether they needed any shaping to maximize their effectiveness.

Common Problems in Solution Evaluation

A variety of problems interfere with effective solution evaluation including failure to conduct any solution evaluation. Though not every solution requires a substantial amount of evaluation, a lack of evaluation leaves clients vulnerable to not solving their problems effectively, abandoning problem solving, and returning to target behaviors as solutions. More often, therapists fail to implement one of the key components of solution evaluation or do not respond strategically when clients' behaviors interfere with the evaluation. The most severe or prevalent problems tend to occur when clients reject solutions without seeming to evaluate them first. Just as therapists sometimes question clients' suggestions for solutions, clients frequently consider therapists' suggestions to be more problematic than useful. Most commonly clients express this opinion with a simple statement such as "That won't work" or "I can't do that." In response, therapists may fail to adequately assess the validity of such statements and make inaccurate assumptions about them. Therapists sometimes automatically accept clients' rejections and consequently miss targeting a TIB and instead reinforce invalid rejecting. Alternatively, therapists mistakenly reject clients' objections and consequently miss identifying valid obstacles and instead invalidate the client. Unfortunately, even when a therapist validates a client's valid objections, the solution evaluation may still go awry if the therapist fails to identify the specific obstacles that will impede implementation or to treat removable obstacles.

Rejecting Clients' Objections to Solutions without Evaluation

Although impulsive or repeated objections may require treatment as TIBs, therapists must guard against automatically dismissing these declarations as TIBs and treating them as such. Not only do such automatic assumptions invalidate the client, they derail the therapy from removing actual obstacles and send the treatment along the wrong track. For example, many therapists skip an evaluation of the rejection and just highlight the pros of using and cons of not using the solution to persuade clients to implement it. This response would succeed if a client rejected a solution due exclusively to insufficient orientation to the solution, but in many instances it is the cons of using a solution that control rejection. Some therapists automatically use cheerleading to convince clients to try the rejected solution. Cheerleading could succeed if a client refused because of self-doubts about using the solution successfully, but self-doubt is only one of many factors contributing to rejection. Occasionally a therapist persists in pushing a particular solution, believing that the client absolutely needs this solution and that with enough persistence the client will agree. Though such persistence sometimes pays, DBT views no single solution as essential and a strong attachment to any specific solution as a possible cause of suffering for therapist and client alike.

Certain factors tend to increase the likelihood of therapists dismissing or minimizing clients' objections. Quite understandably, therapists seem more likely to ignore oversimplified statements such as "That won't work" than specific statements such as "Whenever I try to assert myself, my boyfriend threatens to leave." Alternatively, a therapist might reject "That won't work" because the therapist has remembered the solution working for the client in another context, but has forgotten the possibility of "apparent competence." Similarly, therapists sometimes make assumptions about clients' objections because they know that some client populations have a cognitive bias toward anticipating failure.

Therapists must discriminate between those occasions when clients' rejection of solutions constitutes a valid obstacle and when it constitutes a TIB. In addition to considering the impulsivity and pervasiveness of any rejection, therapists can best assess this distinction by asking for more specificity in response to a general rejection and trying the solution in the session whenever possible. For example, one therapist complained to the consultation team that her client consistently said, "I can't do mindfulness," despite having attended multiple skills training groups on mindfulness. The therapist had tried to treat this behavior by trying "to convince" the client of the benefits of mindfulness and that she could do it if she "just practiced more." The team highlighted that the therapist had not tried, however, to assess the accuracy of the client's statement by having the client try mindfulness during the session. They also highlighted the therapist's assumption that attending skills training leads directly to skills generalization. When the therapist assessed the client's actual ability through in-session practice, they discovered the validity in the client's assertion. Though the client noticed and labeled unmindful thoughts well, the thoughts returned when she tried to "let go" of them, and she genuinely did not know what to do next.

Failing to Evaluate and Treat Specific Obstacles to Implementation

Sometimes a therapist accepts a client's valid objection but then fails to further evaluate or treat the objection and drops the solution too quickly. Though therapists may strategically decide to focus on another solution or another controlling variable, therapists who do so nonstrategically (e.g., because of mindlessness or fear of challenging a client) leave clients handicapped. For example, if a therapist simply accepts a valid "I can't" without understanding exactly what the client cannot do, the therapist will not treat this capability deficit and the client will remain incapable. If Blanche's therapist had simply accepted Blanche's "I can't remember" rather than identifying the specific obstacles to remembering (e.g., a cueing deficit, dysfunctional contingencies), the solution analysis would have depended on environmental interventions only and thus reinforced Blanche's active passivity. In one case, the therapist accepted, without further analysis, the client's statement that the client could not afford to phone the therapist for coaching because he had no money for his phone. When she reviewed her solution analysis with the team, the team suggested that the therapist further assess the client's inability to afford more minutes and troubleshoot this problem, particularly as the client had afforded several drinks with his friends earlier in the day. This analysis revealed that the client could remove the financial obstacle with better budgeting. In several cases, individual therapists have identified a specific skill deficit but have then waited for the skills training group to teach the relevant solution rather than teaching clients themselves. This may prove an efficient strategy if the skill plays a minor role in the solution analysis or the group plans to teach the relevant skill soon. If the solution reappears throughout the analysis or the group will not teach the skill for several months, however, the procrastinating can significantly weaken the solution analysis. DBT requires that individual therapists know how to teach all of the DBT skills as well as skills trainers do.

Accepting Clients' Objections to Solutions without Evaluation

Just as some therapists have rejected clients' valid objections, other therapists have accepted clients' invalid objections and have thus failed to treat a TIB. Accepting an invalid objection often leads the therapist to miss other obstacles to the solution, such as not evaluating clients' capabilities in the situation or missing motivational deficits. Many clients declare that they "can't" do something when they "don't want" to do something. In such cases, an evaluation could reveal not only a general motivational deficit, but also the specific factors that maintain the deficit.

When therapists notice a repetition of invalid objections, it usually proves more efficient to target the pattern of behavior than to treat each objection on its own. In such cases, therapists would employ a brief behavioral chain and solution analysis as they would with other TIBs. For example, when a therapist analyzed one client's pattern of "I can't," she discovered that the behavior functioned to elicit environmental support and that she had reinforced the behavior herself. As a primary solution, she reversed the contingency such that she decreased support in response to rejected solutions and increased support in response to accepted solutions. In particular, she arranged scheduled coaching calls in proportion to the number and difficulty of the solutions that the client agreed to implement.

If a therapist persistently fails to analyze such TIBs, then the consultation team would conduct a brief behavioral chain and solution analysis of the therapist's behavior. For example, when one therapist consistently failed to analyze the client's repeated response of "That won't work," the analysis by the team revealed that the therapist believed that she "shouldn't invalidate" the client and worried how the client would respond to any invalidation. The team challenged the therapist's rule about invalidation and then addressed the worries by role-playing how to challenge the client with maximal effect and minimal conflict and how to resolve any conflict.

SOLUTION IMPLEMENTATION

Conceptualization and Strategies

In comparison to solution generation and evaluation, solution implementation involves more doing than thinking or conceptualizing. The client and therapist first choose a solution to implement. As described in the introduction to solution analysis, therapists encourage clients to choose the solution(s) whenever possible. A therapist might ask, "Which solution will you commit to using?" or "Which solution do you want to practice?" If the therapist believes that the client needs to try more than one solution for a controlling variable, the therapist might ask, "Which solution do you want to rehearse first?" DBT therapists, however, do not ask, "Do you want to try any solutions?"

If the selected solution is either new or a weak response in the client's existing repertoire, the therapy proceeds to implementing the solution during the session whenever possible. Such in-session implementation strengthens skills and challenges clients' expectations of failure. It also allows the therapist and client to identify and remove any obstacles that might interfere with the successful implementation of the skills outside of therapy. Clients may practice letting go of judgments, accepting reality as it is, acting opposite to emotional urges, validating others, or a combination of all of these during a session. With the assistance of their therapists, clients may restructure dysfunctional cognitions and expose themselves to cues that elicit unwarranted emotions while preventing dysfunctional behavioral responses. Therapists may impose new contingencies to shape clients' behaviors or help clients do this for themselves. DBT often implements and interweaves these procedures more informally than traditional CBT does. For example, if a client avoids asking the therapist for help because the client fears that the therapist will respond with rejection, exposure would probably serve as the primary intervention. Rather than constructing a hierarchy of exposure cues, however, the therapist probably would apply exposure to the current context only. In addition, prior to the exposure the therapist might coach the client on relevant interpersonal effectiveness skills training to increase the likelihood that the client will ask for help in a way that the therapist can reinforce. This less formal approach, however, does not mean that therapists forgo all orientation to the essential elements of a solution. For example, when rehearsing interpersonal skills, a therapist might focus the rehearsal on the skills relevant to the identified scenario but prompt the client to rehearse each of those skills (e.g., asserting wants, validating the other person) individually before combining them in a more natural role play.

After the client has implemented the solution, the therapist assesses the client's experience and provides reinforcement and feedback. When necessary, the therapist further shapes the implementation of the solution by addressing any problems that have arisen and trying the solution again. Though the effectiveness of the solution ultimately determines whether clients continue to use it, therapists can also reinforce solution implementation, at least in the therapy context, through their responses. Effective reinforcement requires therapists to assess the reinforcing value of their responses rather than making assumptions about it. For example, praise reinforces some clients, but punishes others; more therapy time rewards some clients but not others. In addition to reinforcing clients' practice generally, therapists also highlight specifically what clients did well and how they can further increase the solution's effectiveness. For example, when Emma first rehearsed using interpersonal skills to reduce domestic demands, her therapist noticed that Emma used the "DEAR MAN GIVE" skills to obtain her objective while maintaining the relationship but that Emma did not use any "FAST" skills to maintain her self-respect. If the client has notable difficulty applying the solution, the therapist would troubleshoot the issue. This occurred when Alexandra finally agreed to rehearse validating her boyfriend. Before agreeing to rehearse validation, she had learned to label "He [her boyfriend] doesn't deserve validation" as a judgment and had worked on letting it go. Unfortunately, when she rehearsed validation, she became repeatedly distracted by the thought. Alexandra reported that she recognized the thought as a judgment, but did not know how to let it go when it seemed so constant. Her therapist then provided detailed coaching on how to refocus her attention and fully participate in rehearsing validation. When solution implementation reviews involve either significant feedback for improvement or significant troubleshooting, the solution will usually require additional in-session application. For example, Emma again rehearsed negotiating for a reduction of domestic demands, but this time with an emphasis on maintaining her self-respect. Alexandra again rehearsed validating her boyfriend, this time mindfully focusing on the task and away from distracting judgments. Usually, practicing a few solutions with such shaping yields better results than practicing many solutions without any shaping.

Finally, if they have not done so earlier, therapists use commitment-strengthening strategies to increase the likelihood that clients will apply the solution outside of the therapy session. Linehan's (1993a) emphasis on commitment derives from social psychology literature, which reveals that using strategies to elicit and strengthen an individual's initial commitment to a behavior significantly increases the likelihood that the behavior will occur. Specific techniques include cheerleading (i.e., expressing confidence in a client's capacity to succeed) and connecting present commitments to prior commitments. Other commitment strategies require the therapist to behave dialectically, such as playing the devil's advocate against a solution and highlighting both the freedom not to use a solution and the absence of alternative solutions.

Common Problems in Solution Implementation

Even if therapists have successfully generated and evaluated solutions, the solution analysis as a whole can falter or even fail because of problems with solution implementation. Common problems include an absence of solution implementation, mistaking minimal for full implementation, insufficiently specifying the essential elements of the solution, not shaping the practice, and reinforcing clients' TIBs.

Failing to Implement Any Solution

The most serious problem is failing to include any solution implementation. Therapists tend to miss solution implementation for the same reasons that they fail to include solution analyses altogether. Fortunately, the same remedies apply. Some therapists simply learn solution analysis one component at a time, with solution implementation as the last component. Other therapists become inhibited when prompting clients to *do* something, rather than just discussing doing something. In such cases, the therapist or consultation team may need to analyze the inhibition and implement solutions for the key controlling variables. For example, one therapist admitted to her team that she avoided implementing key solutions because she "struggled" with shaping mindfulness and feared applying exposure. To solve this issue, the team assigned the therapist

relevant reading, modeled how to shape mindfulness and apply exposure, and then role-played these strategies with the therapist. They also
coached her on which strategies to use if her clients responded poorly.

Failing to Implement Solutions Fully

Therapists often believe that they have fully implemented a solution during a session when they have only summarized or partially implemented
the solution. For example, many therapists believe that they have implemented cognitive restructuring when they have only asked a series of
challenging questions to which the clients have responded with "Yes" or
"No." Such questioning can model one way to restructure cognitions,
but at that point clients have rehearsed only saying "Yes" and "No"
with any certainty. They have not rehearsed cognitive restructuring
themselves, thus reducing the opportunity to shape new behavior and
to identify and treat any obstacles to implementation. Fully implementing this solution during the session requires rehearsal by, not just agreement from, the client. Thus, the therapist might say, "So next time you
have that thought, what are you going to say to yourself to change it?"
In addition to mistaking modeling for fully implementing a solution,
therapists sometimes confuse summarizing with practicing. For example, summarizing or listing relevant "DEAR MAN" interpersonal skills
does not equate to rehearsing them in a session. To practice these skills,
the client and therapist need to role-play them in a relevant scenario,
with the client actually saying what he or she plans to say outside of the
therapy session.

Failing to Specify the Solution's Essential Elements

Frequently, clients struggle or fail to implement a solution successfully,
either during or after a session, because their therapists have not specified or structured the essential elements of the solution sufficiently. For
example, many clients struggle to practice mindfulness because their
therapists have not reviewed the required components. One therapist
asked the consultation team for help with a client who reported that her
judgmental thoughts returned whenever they practiced being nonjudgmental. While listening to a recording of the session, the team noticed
that in structuring the practice, the therapist reminded the client to label
judgmental thoughts but did not include any additional steps. The team
then role-played with the therapist how to give the client instructions
first to describe the facts of the situation and then to participate in the
task at hand. When the therapist implemented this consultation, the

client reported that the judgments subsided better if she noticed them and then returned her attention to the task of the moment. Similarly, when another therapist reported that "acting opposite" did not decrease her client's unwarranted shame, the consultation team listened to the relevant recording and discovered that the therapist had not instructed the client to act opposite to all elements of the emotion. When the therapist reviewed each element with the client, they discovered that the client previously had not acted opposite to her shaming body posture and cognitions.

Not Shaping Implementation

Therapists sometimes effectively encourage clients to implement a solution during the session, but then do not adequately shape the implementation. Though therapists may decide to forgo shaping for strategic reasons (e.g., efficiency), they often fail to provide constructive feedback because they did not notice subtle issues, did not know how to address the issues, or became inhibited about addressing them. When implementing exposure, for example, some therapists focus on blocking obvious overt behaviors and miss more subtle facial, postural, or verbal behaviors. Similarly, when clients have used "DEAR MAN" skills competently in a role play but have not demonstrated the necessary "GIVE" skills, some therapists praise the former but fail to provide feedback and coaching on the latter. Alternatively, therapists may notice opportunities to shape a skill but they fear that any critical feedback will upset clients and so do not provide the feedback. To resolve these issues, therapists can analyze and treat them with the consultation team, but the more subtle aspects of some of these issues may require a review of actual session recordings. Finally, though the successful implementation of a solution may require no more feedback than a "Well done," clients often find a more detailed description of what they did well to be more helpful, more reinforcing, or both.

Client-Interfering Behaviors

As with the other components of solution generation, clients engage in a variety of behaviors that interfere with solution implementation. These behaviors include refusing to implement a solution, not fully participating in the implementation, and committing only to "trying" outside of the session. Ironically, therapists sometimes inadvertently prompt some of these behaviors when they prioritize polite speech over clear instructions. If a therapist thinks that a client needs to rehearse a skill but instead "politely" asks, "Do you want to practice this skill?" then the client may respond honestly rather than helpfully with "No." The question does not ask what the therapist genuinely wants to know and it directs clients to attend to doing what they want rather than what will be effective. DBT highlights the importance of therapists being genuine and focusing on effectiveness in their communication with clients. Although therapists can quickly correct problematic prompts, they risk creating a bigger problem if they reinforce rather than treat clients' TIBs. For example, one therapist accepted an "I'll try" as a sufficient commitment, but the client did not fully implement the solution during the week. When the same pattern occurred the following week, the therapist expressed her frustration about the client "not keeping commitments to using solutions" to the consultation team. The team highlighted that the therapist had only obtained a commitment to "trying" and suggested that the therapist might have reinforced the client's avoidance of committing to the solution. The team then role-played commitment-strengthening strategies so that the therapist could treat rather than reinforce the problem. Often, the treatment of clients' behaviors that interfere with implementation requires nothing more than blocking those behaviors or applying solutions that have worked with other TIBs. At other times, the treatment will require a brief BCA and solution analysis. For example, when Jack (the inpatient disliked by staff) refused to rehearse interpersonal skills and added "They're stupid," his therapist initially tried to increase Jack's motivation by linking the skill to his goals. Jack still refused, and the therapist then realized that they needed to analyze what controlled the refusal. The analysis revealed that Jack already understood the utility of the solution, but that he anticipated "getting it wrong" during the rehearsal and felt notably embarrassed. Refusing to practice and labeling the skills as "stupid" functioned to decrease the embarrassment by dissuading the therapist from pursuing the rehearsal. When the therapist offered Jack the choice of first treating the anticipating or the embarrassment, Jack chose the anticipating. They decided to select mindfulness as a solution, particularly focusing on the moment and letting go of judgments. They then progressed to treating the embarrassment and decided to use acting opposite to the emotion, as the context did not warrant such intense embarrassment. They first focused on acting opposite to the postural and verbal elements of the emotion. In particular, the therapist had Jack act opposite to his refusal to rehearse by asking to rehearse the interpersonal skills. Finally, Jack rehearsed the interpersonal skills.

CHAPTER 5

SKILLS TRAINING

Skills training has become the solution most associated with DBT. As described in Chapter 1, recent research (Neacsiu, Rizvi, & Linehan, 2010) validates the inclusion of skills training as a critical component of DBT. A separate skills training treatment manual (Linehan, 1993b, 2014), complete with lecture and discussion points, handouts, and homework assignments, describes the implementation of skills training as a solution. Sometimes, however, therapists confuse skills training with simply working through the skills training. Therapists may assume, for example, that learning a new skill simply requires that the therapist present the lecture points, handouts, and worksheets for that new skill. By oversimplifying the process of implementing new skills, therapists inadvertently invalidate their clients, much as clients' original invalidating environments did.

Linehan (1993a, 1993b) describes three basic procedures required for successful skills training: (1) skills acquisition, (2) skills strengthening, and (3) skills generalization. In skills acquisition, therapists inform clients about the new skill by orienting them to the skill's purpose, instructing them about its core components or steps and modeling how to implement the skill. During skills strengthening, clients practice the new skill and therapists then reinforce any skill use. Therapists then provide corrective feedback and coaching to further shape the skill. Finally, skills generalization requires therapists to assist clients in implementing new skills and integrating multiple skills in all relevant contexts. DBT requires that providers in all DBT treatment modalities have the capacity to apply all of these training procedures. For example, although DBT programs expect the group skills trainers to provide skills acquisition for all of the skills, individual therapists often need to implement this procedure with their own clients because the group has not yet taught the skill the client needs now or because a client missed the relevant group session. Skills coaches primarily focus on generalization procedures, but their sessions often involve skills strengthening. Thus, during their DBT training, all therapists, not just skills trainers, need to read the skills training manual (Linehan, 1993b, 2014), practice all of the skills, and complete all of the corresponding homework. This process will provide them with at least some experience of the three skills training procedures, as well as knowledge about each skill. This chapter focuses on the principles, strategies, and common problems for each type of skills training procedure.

Although skills deficits are central to the DBT conceptualization of BPD, the treatment modalities differ in the extent to which they assess skills deficits, teach skills as solutions, and exclusively teach DBT skills. For example, group skills trainers determine in advance which DBT skill(s) they will teach each week without first assessing whether each group client lacks that skill(s). They then focus the session on training the DBT skill(s), with time allocated for each type of skills procedure. In contrast, individual therapists have no predetermined skills training agenda. During the course of solution analysis the therapist and client decide which skills would help to solve the problem. The solution analysis need not rely on DBT skills alone. For example, one therapist had to teach her client interview skills to help the client obtain a job. Another therapist had to teach the client basic financial planning skills to help the client reduce debt. The individual therapist and client must also determine whether the lack of skill use resulted from a skills deficit versus a motivational deficit. A skills deficit can result from a lack of skills acquisition, strengthening, or generalization. To assess for deficits, the therapist may ask the client directly whether he or she knows the skill and about what interfered with using it. Furthermore, therapists observe clients' skill use within the therapy context and ask them to demonstrate relevant skills. These assessment methods generally work best in combination, as singularly they can produce misleading results. For example, many clients will say, "I can't use the skill," which would lead to skills training, when a more thorough assessment reveals that they lack sufficient motivation to implement the skill. Similarly, failure to observe the skill occurring naturalistically does not necessarily indicate that a client lacks the capacity, as other variables (e.g., emotions, cognition, or contingencies) may inhibit the client from using the skill. Fortunately, assuming a capability deficit and teaching a specific skill only to discover that the client actually does possess the skill causes far fewer problems than assuming that the client *does* have the skill when in fact he or she does not. If in the middle of teaching a new skill the therapist discovers that the client already has the skill, the therapist would then begin to analyze the factors that interfered with the use of the skill. The clinical examples in this chapter derive primarily from experiences in which the therapist and client have identified a DBT skill deficit from one of the standard DBT skills modules (i.e., mindfulness, emotion regulation, distress tolerance, or interpersonal effectiveness).

Skills trainers and individual therapists also differ with respect to when and how they address clients' TIBs. Because skills trainers have the responsibility to teach as much about the skills as possible to as many clients as possible, they cannot stop the entire skills training process to assess and develop a treatment plan for the behavior of a single client every time a TIB occurs. Although skills trainers intervene immediately to stop any behavior that threatens to destroy therapy and have time reserved during the homework review to treat not completing homework, they might have only a brief opportunity to target other TIBs. Sometimes just blocking or highlighting a behavior, clarifying or applying a few contingencies, or suggesting a few skills suffices to solve the problem. If not, skills trainers may further target the behavior during breaks or after the group. If the behavior persists, skills trainers will refer the client to the individual therapist, who has the primary responsibility for treating all of a client's TIBs, for a more comprehensive analysis.

In Max's case, his skills trainers noticed that he seemed to struggle to remember what they had taught in class from week to week and that he frequently spent time looking toward the window. They hypothesized a connection between these behaviors but did not have a chance to analyze what controlled the "not remembering." They called his name whenever they noticed him looking toward the window, which temporarily reoriented his attention, and encouraged him to take notes during group. When the "not remembering" continued, they encouraged Max to tell his therapist and shared their observations with the consultation team. Max reported to his therapist that he frequently did not remember what had been taught in skills group. A BCA of not remembering parts of the last skills session established that the focus on an interpersonal skill in that session had elicited ruminations about how past relationships had gone awry, which then led to judgments and worry thoughts that then cued anxiety, all of which distracted his attention away from the class, thus preventing him from learning the new skill rather than learning and then forgetting it. The therapist and Max then conducted a solution analysis for the most relevant links. Most directly related to Max's attention and his therapist coached him on how to mindfully focus his attention on the session (e.g., looking intently at the skills trainer, looking at the relevant handout, and taking notes, as well as letting go of judgmental and ruminative thoughts). They also agreed that Max would ask the skills trainers to either tap him gently on the arm or ask him a question about the topic in the group if they noticed Max appearing distracted. Implementing these solutions improved Max's capacity to absorb information in the skills group and later proved helpful when he returned to school.

SKILLS ACQUISITION

Conceptualization and Strategies

Orient to the Skill

The basic task in skills acquisition is to provide clients with enough information about a skill to implement it. Clinicians usually begin skills acquisition, as with other change procedures, by orienting clients to the skill, including its primary function and expected impact. For example, if Rita had not previously received an orientation to the interpersonal effectiveness "GIVE" skill during her skills training class, her therapist would have oriented her to it during the course of writing an apology to the psychiatrist. The orientation would have clarified that the "GIVE" skill would assist Rita to repair her relationship with the psychiatrist and likely increase the psychiatrist's motivation to collaborate with her. Similarly, had Susan not learned about the emotion regulation skill of "opposite action" in skills class, her therapist would have clarified that the skill would function to decrease the unwarranted intensity of her guilt and shame by changing the behaviors associated with the emotions. Orienting to skills also often involves clarifying what not to expect from skills. For example, although mindfulness skills frequently decrease negative emotions, they do not function primarily to regulate emotions; clinicians should discourage clients from assessing the effectiveness of the skills or their success in implementing them based on whether negative emotions cease. Similarly, the interpersonal skills generally increase the likelihood of achieving an interpersonal goal, but they do not guarantee success.

Provide Didactic Information

After orientation, clinicians provide clear, didactic information about the behavioral components involved in the skill, as described in the skills training manual (Linehan, 1993b, 2014). These behavioral instructions range from general guidelines to specific instructions. For example, when Jane learned about opposite action in skills training class, she learned about the different components of emotions (e.g., facial expression, body posture, cognitions, impulses) to which she needed to attend when acting opposite. She also learned how to act opposite to the components, but she did not receive specific instructions about how to implement the skills when experiencing intense guilt and shame after arguing with her mother and not fitting into her jeans. Her individual therapist, however, gave specific suggestions for the various components that they identified during the BCA. The therapist instructed her to hold her head up rather than holding it in her hands, walk away from the toilet rather than toward it, and stop ruminating by focusing on the present, specifically on how she could repair the damage done by the argument.

Providing general information about and specific instructions for a skill often necessitates clarifying what the skill does not involve. For example, opposite action does not include masking emotions. One client revealed such a misunderstanding by describing the skill as literally having to "grin and bear" her emotions. Another client expressed a similar belief by describing the skill as "pretending like it doesn't bother me." Similarly, clinicians often need to clarify that "radical acceptance" does not imply agreeing with or acquiescing to a situation. Clients may indicate such an assumption by using the phrase "I've just *got* to accept it," a phrase commonly used to describe a willpower-based approach to life's vicissitudes. This phrasing implies the absence of choice, a moral imperative, or a tacit "should" to accept whatever the circumstances. None of this represents the essence of radical acceptance. Using radical acceptance requires intentionally choosing to turn toward the situation rather than turning away and not radically accepting.

Clients also often have inaccurate assumptions about how quickly and dramatically a skill will work and how much effort and perseverance it requires. For example, many clients anticipate that opposite action will instantly decrease emotional intensity from high to none. Many also expect that noticing a ruminative thought and returning their attention to the present once will stop all ruminative thinking in the situation. Though many factors contribute to clients' erroneous expectations, individual therapists ultimately have the responsibility for detecting, clarifying, and correcting these beliefs.

Model the Skill

In association with didactic instruction, DBT therapists use modeling or demonstrations of the skills. Bandura, the most influential figure in the conceptualization and investigation of modeling, defines a model as "any stimulus array so organized that an observer can extract an act upon the main information conveyed by environmental events without needing to first perform overtly" (Rosenthal & Bandura, 1978, p. 3). Modeling can serve various functions, but in relation to skills acquisition it refers to the "learning of a novel sequence of behavior as a result of observing a model" (Wilson & O'Leary, 1980, p. 188). During sessions, for example, therapists demonstrate the skill through role plays, tell teaching stories, or show video clips. They may also encourage clients to observe other appropriate models outside of therapy, in either the clients' natural environments or through the media, such as public figures on television, historical figures in biographies, and fictional characters in literature or on film. For example, the Agatha Christie Poirot mysteries and similar types of detective fiction consistently illustrate how to mindfully observe and how to differentiate observing from interpreting or being judgmental. Biographies or documentaries of Nelson Mandela provide multiple examples of radical acceptance. The film *Groundhog Day* illustrates how interpersonal skills sometimes require practice and shaping again and again and again before they become effective. In addition to providing information, demonstrations and other types of modeling appear particularly effective at engaging clients' attention, a key factor in successful skills acquisition.

Like most behavioral treatments, DBT emphasizes coping rather than mastery models. More than most therapies, DBT encourages therapists to use self-disclosure as a coping model (Linehan, 1993a). For example, part of Jane's repair to her mother involved using the "GIVE" interpersonal skills, both to apologize in general and to assess and repair the damage done to her mother and their relationship in particular. To help Jane acquire the required skills, her therapist described to Jane how she had used the "GIVE" skills with her own mother following a recent argument. Though Jane found the modeling of the skills themselves quite helpful, she found her therapist's modeling of how to manage difficulties in skill implementation even more useful. Another client said that what she had learned most from her therapist's self-disclosure of mindfulness as a solution for rumination and anger was how much persistence it required and how to notice that she had become unmindful "again." In addition to describing skills used in daily life, therapists demonstrate the use of skills, especially mindfulness, within sessions. For example, therapists notice their own judgments or assumptions, comment aloud on this, and describe the skill they use to counteract the problem. In one case, when a client told the therapist that her father had described her on the Internet as a crack whore, the therapist initially responded by being judgmental of the father. She then said, "But I'm being judgmental and that isn't going to help you decide how to respond to the message or those who say something about it. I'm going to let go of the judgments and focus on helping you solve the problem." This entire response created a dialectical balance in the session in which the client experienced the validation of the therapist's radical genuineness and the modeling of noticing judgments, letting them go, and focusing on the task at hand. Therapists can increase their ability to apply self-disclosure by practicing all of the skills and completing all of the homework described in the skills training manual (Linehan, 1993b, 2014) during their training or early implementation of the therapy.

Common Problems

Problems with skills acquisition occur most frequently in skills training classes and individual therapy, as telephone coaching and related modalities usually focus on generalizing skills that the client has already acquired. Some problems occur more frequently in one modality or the other. For example, failing to teach a relevant skill at all occurs almost exclusively in individual therapy, as skills trainers have an a priori plan to teach specific skills each week. Many problems, however, seem to appear with similar frequency in both settings. These include providing inaccurate information about the function or components of a skill, failing to provide sufficient information about the components of the skill, and oversimplifying the difficulty of learning a new skill.

Failing to Teach a Critical Skill

Sometimes individual therapists generate a skill as part of the solution analysis but fail to provide any skills acquisition, even when clients lack basic knowledge of the skill and the skill has a critical role in the solution analysis. In some instances, therapists omit skills acquisition because they do not know enough about the skill to teach someone else. This seems to happen more often with therapists who have little or no experience as a DBT skills trainer. Teaching a skills training class generally necessitates sufficient preparation to ensure that therapists know at least some of the basic points, and answering group members' questions further refines this knowledge. Furthermore, listening to clients share their experience with skills practice gives therapists valuable feedback about how well they taught the skill. If a therapist cannot participate in a skills training class, watching a skills training video or role-playing teaching the skill during consultation meetings can provide the therapist with sufficient knowledge. In other cases, therapists make a strategic decision not to use time during their sessions to teach clients a skill that the skills trainers will eventually teach. Though this can prove an efficient strategy for skills that have less importance in the solution analysis, applying this strategy to critical skills could prolong a client's suffering for weeks or even months.

To teach clients a new skill efficiently during individual sessions, therapists extract the essential elements from the skill and focus on teaching clients what they need to know about the skill to use it in just the context of the current solution analysis. For example, rather than lecturing at length about opposite action in general or providing detailed information about how to apply it to every emotion, the therapist would provide a brief orientation to the skill generally and then focus on how exactly to act opposite to the emotion as it occurred in that context. Finally, therapists who miss skills acquisition often do so because they assume that clients learned the basics of the skill in class. High apparent competence in clients can increase the likelihood of this occurring. A tendency by therapists to minimize the difficulty of learning new skills also seems related to making this assumption. Assessing a client's knowledge of a new skill whenever the skill is first included in a solution analysis will help to minimize any inaccurate assumptions.

Providing Inaccurate Information about a Skill

Significant problems occur if either the skills trainers or the individual therapist provide inaccurate information about a skill, including its function, likely consequences or components, or if they fail to correct a client's misunderstanding. For example, some trainers and therapists have taught clients that opposite action requires them to act in a way that elicits an opposite emotion rather than simply acting opposite to the covert and overt behaviors associated with the existing emotion. Skills trainers can obtain corrective feedback from each other, unless they share the same inaccurate beliefs, and individual therapists can give skills trainers feedback if they discover during individual therapy that the client has received incorrect information from skills trainers. Listening to recordings of therapy sessions usually provides the best opportunities for consultation teams to identify when individual therapists have these problems, though role playing may prove a helpful alternative or addition. Usually providing the clinician with corrective feedback and requiring the clinician to rehearse teaching the skill will suffice to solve the problem. If not, the clinician might need to read more extensively (e.g., mindfulness books, articles or chapters on emotion regulation), watch skills training videos, attend relevant trainings (e.g., mindfulness retreats), or practice teaching the skill more during consultation meetings.

As a set, the mindfulness skills seem most vulnerable to errors in clinician teaching and client understanding. Many clinicians have had minimal training in mindfulness, which may partially account for the difficulties. For example, while providing mindfulness instructions, some clinicians confuse "letting go of" with "pushing away" thoughts or emotions. In other instances they have taught clients to believe that mindfulness functions primarily to facilitate relaxation or elicit enjoyment. A clinician might do this directly (e.g., by stating that mindfulness will help clients to relax) or indirectly (e.g., by asking whether clients enjoyed a mindfulness exercise). Mindfulness, however, involves developing a greater awareness of whatever is occurring in the present moment in a nonjudgmental way. Often what is occurring is difficult, distressing, and anything but relaxing. Acknowledging and accepting the distress or discomfort is part of the essence of mindfulness. Clients who expect to "enjoy" mindfulness or "feel relaxed" but then do not have such experiences usually conclude that either mindfulness "doesn't work" or that they "can't do it right." Even for clinicians with experience in other mindfulness-based interventions, problems may arise, as DBT teaches mindfulness in a particular way (Williams & Swales, 2004). For example, many clinicians confuse "being judgmental" as described in the skills training manual with the way that other psychological models use the term "judgment" as a synonym for interpretations (e.g., "He didn't speak to me because he doesn't like me") or expectations (e.g., "None of the skills will work for me"). Although clients often benefit from mindfully noticing, labeling, and letting go of these other types of thoughts, a lack of clarity about judgments and the skill of being nonjudgmental confuses clients at the least and often invalidates the valid.

Some clinicians confuse mindfulness exercises with mindful living. Consequently, clients then believe that mindfulness involves stopping whatever they were doing and doing mindfulness exercises instead. For example, when an individual therapist asked a client to describe mindfulness, the client said, "It's when you're upset, and you rub lotion on your hands and smell it or eat a raisin and pay attention to how it tastes or look at the marks on a leaf." Clients then learn to use mindfulness practices as another way to distract from their lives.

Mindfulness exercises or practices in DBT are just that, exercises or practices designed to teach and strengthen mindfulness skills, similar to how a student completes math exercises or a musician practices chords. The exercises simply provide discrete opportunities to notice the mind wandering and return it to the present moment, to notice judgments or attachments that interfere with acting on the facts of the situation, and to observe an emotion without then acting impulsively. In one case, a therapist noticed that his client frequently came to sessions highly agitated, worrying about a multitude of the events of the past week, and talking rapidly about her worries on entering the therapy room. The therapist correctly identified that the client was unmindful and reasonably decided to intervene to focus the client on the immediate tasks of the session. The therapist suggested that the client practice mindfulness of sounds in the room. The client engaged with the practice and seemed momentarily less agitated but then immediately began listing out her worries as she had before. The failure of the intervention sufficiently surprised the therapist for him to discuss the problem with his team. The team generated two hypotheses. First, the client's emotional arousal may have prevented full participation in the practice, although the momentary cessation in the listing of worries argued against this hypothesis. Second, the client may have used the mindfulness practice as a distraction from the therapy, so that when the distraction ended the unmindful thinking and corresponding behavior returned. After choosing the second hypothesis as more accurate, the therapist and team role-played giving the client behaviorally specific instructions about how to be mindful in the session. Most importantly in this case, the therapist gave directions about how to participate mindfully in the session tasks, specifically to notice when worry thoughts distracted from the task and to re-focus her attention on completing each task, such as answering the therapist's questions, providing information relevant to the task, or implementing a solution. The instructions also included directions to notice the worry and agitation and associated behaviors, including shallow breathing and listing worries, as a first step toward managing the agitation. Providing the client with these instructions about how to be mindful in the existing situation notably increased the client's ability to participate mindfully during the next session.

Neglecting to Teach Components of a Skill

Clinicians sometimes provide accurate information about a new skill, but fail to teach its core components, provide sufficient instructions about them, or model them. For example, clinicians may teach clients how to apply radical acceptance to an event or a situation, but fail to teach clients how to use the skill to cope with their emotional response to the situation or how to accept that if they want to change the situation or their emotional response to it they will need to change their own behavior. This type of problem usually occurs because the clinician lacks sufficient knowledge about the skill or has minimized the difficulty or complexity of acquiring the skill. For example, one individual therapist repeatedly did not model how clients could implement the DBT interpersonal skills because the therapist recognized the inadequacy of his DBT skills knowledge and feared that modeling would expose his ignorance. Clinicians who learn about mindfulness only through the skills manual (Linehan, 1993b) seem less likely to teach clients how to notice other types of unmindful thinking. In numerous instances, clinicians have simply given clients instructions to "notice your judgments and let them go" without providing instructions about how to do this. Thus when clients try to let go of thoughts they either do not succeed at all or the thought returns quickly to "fill the mental void." The solutions described above for communicating inaccurate information equally apply to this problem of communicating incomplete information.

SKILLS STRENGTHENING

Conceptualization and Strategies

Skills strengthening functions to increase the likelihood of clients using identified skills and to enhance the competency with which they use those skills. Skills strengthening procedures in DBT consist of prompting the client to rehearse the skill, reinforcing the clients' skillful rehearsal, providing feedback regarding any problems with the rehearsal, and coaching the client about how to improve implementation of the skill. Bandura (1971) himself proposed that modeling would benefit if followed with practice by the client and then shaping of the practice by the therapist. Subsequent research has consistently validated this proposition. Skills trainers and individual therapists apply skills strengthening procedures any time they introduce clients to a new skill. Skills trainers usually repeat this procedure for a specific skill only when they teach that skill again in class, except for mindfulness skills, which they attempt to strengthen weekly by starting class with a mindfulness exercise. In contrast, individual therapists and skills coaches may need to repeat the procedures multiple times for a skill, even when clients have already acquired basic knowledge about the skill, if the client reveals poor competence with the skill or uses it less frequently than needed.

Behavioral rehearsal requires that clients practice the relevant components of the skill during the session. For example, Jane's therapist requested that Jane rehearse aloud the mindful thoughts that she would generate the next time she thought "I'll always be fat." To rehearse acting opposite to the unwarranted levels of guilt and shame, she had Jane practice lifting her head and making eye contact each time she looked away in the session due to experiencing unwarranted guilt or shame. She also had Jane imagine herself in that situation again and then lifting her head, saying "Stop!" to herself as she approached the toilet and turning away. In contrast, Jack, the inpatient introduced in Chapter 4, and his therapist acted through a situation in which unwarranted anger led him to yell at a nurse who had confronted him about spitting. The therapist played the nurse and Jack played himself using opposite action skills. Jack practiced sitting down rather than approaching the "nurse" and unclenching his hands rather than clenching them into a fist. He also practiced acknowledging responsibility and apologizing in a moderate voice rather than blaming and judging in a loud voice. Susan and her therapist also used role play, in this case to rehearse the interpersonal skills that Susan would use to insist that a male stranger leave her home. When rehearsing more complex skills, clients often need to rehearse the components of the skill separately. For example, Jack and his therapist first rehearsed sitting and unclenching and then rehearsed verbally accepting responsibility and apologizing before combining the components in a role play. As discussed in Chapter 4, therapists must ensure that clients practice the essential elements of the skills rather than just listing them. Also as indicated in Chapter 4, individual therapists must spend more time with newer clients on skills acquisition and strengthening. As therapy progresses and clients have more skills within their repertoires, a smaller subset will necessitate in-session rehearsal.

Although clients must ultimately receive reinforcement for a skill in their natural environment for the skill to maintain a sufficiently high position in the behavioral response hierarchy, clinicians usually need to reinforce skills rehearsal during the learning process for the skill to even appear in the hierarchy. Clinicians provide reinforcement for both practicing generally and for competently demonstrating components of the skill specifically. Though group skills trainers usually do not have enough time to assess exactly what type of response will reinforce each client, individual therapists can maximize the effectiveness and efficiency of their responses by taking time to assess with clients which types of therapist responses will reinforce skills use, as well as those that will punish skills use. Early in treatment, DBT clinicians may offer the only source of contingent reinforcement for skills practice, as clients usually do not find rehearsal itself inherently reinforcing and do not have enough competence in the skill for it to immediately have the intended internal or external effect. As clients engage in rehearsal more consistently and implement skills more competently, therapists fade reinforcement to levels similar to non-DBT environments. Chapter 8 discusses key principles of reinforcement in greater detail.

In addition to using behavioral rehearsal as an opportunity to reinforce competent skill practice, clinicians use rehearsal to identify and correct any errors or omissions in clients' general understanding of or specific attempt at the skill. Identifying errors and omissions necessitates that therapists remain equally alert to verbal and nonverbal behavior and notice subtle aspects of either. For example, one therapist noticed when one client practiced radical acceptance she said, "I radically accept the situation I'm in" while tensing her jaw and clenching her fists. She thus engaged in verbal behavior consistent with the skill, but her nonverbal behavior indicated the contrary. During Jack's first role play the therapist noticed that when Jack sat in the chair he leaned his body forward in a way consistent with preparing to lunge forward and when he apologized his lip curled in a manner that resembled a snarl. If therapists notice an omission or error, they then offer behaviorally specific feedback about the problem and instructions about how to improve implementation. For example, the therapist above described the client's tensed jaw and clenched fists and suggested that the client might find radical acceptance more effective if she changed these. The therapist then provided specific instructions about how to use her body as part of the skill. Jack's therapist modeled several ways to sit in the chair that would block "lunging" forward. Ideally, after the feedback and coaching therapists will ask clients to rehearse the skill again. Jack required three role plays before the skill seemed strong enough for him to have even a chance of implementing it successfully on the unit. Therapists often can improve the efficiency of skills strengthening procedures by interrupting clients' rehearsals as soon as they notice an error, especially if they have previously provided feedback and coaching about that error. When Jack lunged forward during the second role play, his therapist stopped the role play, provided some praise, and then requested that Jack simply practice different ways of sitting that would block lunging before they returned to the role play as a whole. During both the second and third role plays, whenever Jack curled his lip, the therapist provided feedback by simply saying "Uncurl," which prompted Jack to implement the relevant instructions. Such interruptions block the potential for reinforcement of errors, though therapists must check that they do not punish trying to rehearse the skill as well. Successfully providing feedback and coaching also necessitates knowing how much feedback will overwhelm or discourage a client.

Common Problems

A variety of problems can occur with respect to skills strengthening procedures. Failing to rehearse skills at all is the most significant problem among individual therapists, though it occurs less often in skills training as the skills manual (Linehan, 1993b, 2014) contains specific instructions about when and what to rehearse. Problematic behaviors that occur across modalities include not rehearsing skills sufficiently, reinforcing clients' refusal to or avoidance of rehearsing, failing to provide needed feedback and coaching, providing erroneous feedback, and oversimplifying the skill when offering coaching. Many of the solutions described in Chapter 4 for solution implementation apply to problems in skills strengthening.

Failing to Request Skill Rehearsal

Clinicians vary in their ability to recognize whether they repeatedly skip behavioral rehearsal or accept only perfunctory practice. Skills trainers have the advantage of working with co-trainers who might notice a problem that the other has missed. Some individual therapists and skills coaches identify the problem themselves, but others gain awareness only after the consultation team has listened to a recording or conducted a role play with the therapist. Similarly, some clinicians easily identify the reasons for the problem, whereas others require a more structured analysis of the controlling variables. As discussed in Chapter 4 on solution analysis, common reasons include poor time management, a belief in or preference for insight over action, and confusion between describing or summarizing a skill and rehearsing it. Cognitions and emotions, warranted or unwarranted, often inhibit requesting skills rehearsal. For example, many therapists may fear that clients will refuse and the therapist will not know how to respond to the clients' TIBs. Some therapists feel guilt about asking clients to do something difficult, and a few experience embarrassment themselves while role-playing.

In some instances, clinicians can generate and implement solutions for rehearsal problems with little or no consultation from the team. For example, some individual therapists have reported that simply spending a period of time as skills trainers significantly helped to address a variety of reasons for the problem. A therapist who does not know how to respond to clients' refusals to rehearse may ask the team to role-play various options. In one case, the therapist identified two key controlling variables for minimizing behavioral rehearsal, namely, the thought that "Rehearsing makes no difference, as my client doesn't use the skills anyway," and the fact that her client seldom did implement new skills. For the thought, she tried cognitive restructuring and mindfully not attending to it, focusing instead on fully participating in the behavioral rehearsal. In this instance, the mindfulness proved more effective, as cognitive restructuring distracted her from rehearsal for longer. For the absence of reinforcement she sought consultation from the team about how to increase the client's skills use. The team provided consultation, but anticipated that the skills use would improve slowly, so they suggested that the therapist also focus on other immediate reinforcement for rehearsing with the client. The therapist discovered that evaluating her own performance in terms of her treatment adherence rather than the client's skills use notably increased the reinforcement for rehearsing.

In some cases, clinicians may need more consultation from the team to identify causal variables leading to the rehearsal problem or more assistance in implementing relevant solutions. In one case, the team initially identified cognitions related to minimizing the impact of skills rehearsal as the main reason that the therapist seldom asked clients to rehearse. They attempted to use cognitive restructuring by presenting relevant data, as well as suggesting mindfulness of the interfering cognitions. When the therapist's behavior failed to improve, a new analysis of the problem revealed that the therapist usually "felt tired" during sessions and wanted to minimize his efforts and that the cognitions functioned to justify making less effort. The team then focused its solution analysis on the "tiredness" and attended to managing contingencies for conducting adherent therapy versus minimizing efforts. In another case, the therapist knew that embarrassment inhibited her from doing role plays in any therapeutic context and that this interfered with both her modeling of and the client's rehearsal of interpersonal skills. She decided to try opposite action by asking the consultation team to "require" weekly interpersonal role plays from her. During these role plays, the team identified several embarrassment-related behaviors, including the hesitant way in which the therapist requested the "client" to rehearse, her body posture during the rehearsal, and her extensive and overgeneral praise of the "client" at the end. Over time, however, her role playing during sessions did not increase, nor did her embarrassment decrease. An analysis by the team revealed that although the therapist had overtly acted opposite, covertly she had maintained several embarrassment-related cognitions, particularly chronic and negative self-appraisals. Her embarrassment decreased only after the therapist treated these cognitions with mindfulness.

Reinforcing Clients' Refusals to Rehearse

Some therapists adherently request behavioral rehearsal during a session but then reinforce clients refusing or otherwise avoiding rehearsal. Such reinforcement may result from therapists colluding with clients because of therapists' own motivational issues, in which previously discussed strategies for motivational variables apply. Alternatively, therapists may have a skills deficit regarding more strategic responses. In these cases, therapists need to learn and apply the same types of problem-solving strategies as they would to any other client TIB. On many occasions simply reminding clients briefly about their goals and linking those goals directly to the skills practice can suffice. Similarly, clarifying other contingencies of refusing can reduce avoidance enough. For example, after Rita and her therapist discussed which interpersonal skills to use instead of threatening the psychiatrist (see Box 4.1 in Chapter 4), Rita initially refused. Her therapist then highlighted that rehearsing the skills in session probably would increase Rita's ability to use them later with the psychiatrist and consequently to achieve her interpersonal goals, namely, for the psychiatrist to "understand" her and not to discharge her. The therapist also clarified that Rita's continued refusal would decrease her own motivation to help Rita manage her relationship with the psychiatrist. Rita then agreed to rehearse, albeit reluctantly at first. On other occasions, clients will stop refusing if their therapists briefly coach them on how to decrease or tolerate any emotion controlling the refusal.

If such brief interventions fail, then the therapist would progress to conducting a brief but more structured BCA of the factors resulting in the refusal. In the case of Janine, an inpatient with anorexia, the consultation team noticed while listening to a session recording that the therapist always moved immediately to another solution if she asked Janine to rehearse a solution and Janine refused. The therapist explained that in response to previous rehearsals, she had linked the rehearsal to Janine's goals and clarified the benefits of rehearsing and costs of not rehearsing, but Janine had always continued to refuse. The team highlighted that the therapist had only tried to "talk the client into" rehearsing and had never analyzed why Janine refused. During the next individual therapy session, when Janine refused to rehearse describing her body mindfully rather than judgmentally, the therapist conducted a brief analysis of the refusal. She discovered that following the request Janine anticipated focusing on her body and immediately experienced intense physical disgust. Next, she then thought her therapist "shouldn't ask me to do this. She knows it will make me vomit," and experienced a surge of anger that led to a decrease in the disgust and refusing to rehearse. The disgust then decreased further, and Janine revealed that in the past when the therapist had stopped asking for rehearsal, the anger had dissipated as well. Following this analysis, the therapist validated Jane's reluctance, particularly because the request to practice provoked such distressing emotions and because refusal had previously been reinforced by the reduction in both emotional distress and therapist requests for rehearsal. They then agreed to focus on treating the disgust, as the anger seemed like a secondary emotion that functioned to facilitate avoidance of the disgust.

Janine willingly rehearsed various aspects of opposite action to reduce the disgust, including moving forward rather than pressing back against the chair, looking forward rather than turning her head away, opening her eyes instead of squinting, relaxing her nose rather than wrinkling it, and half smiling instead of tensing her upper lip. Janine also rehearsed radical acceptance of experiencing some disgust. With some hesitation the therapist then asked Janine again to rehearse describing her body mindfully, and Janine agreed, using opposite action to minimize the disgust that the rehearsal initially elicited. This return to the original request that elicited the refusal was essential to the treatment of the TIB. Without it, the analysis of the refusal to rehearse could have served as further avoidance of the necessary practice. In other words, the therapist used contingency management procedures to combat the historical avoidance of rehearsal.

Neglecting to Provide Feedback and Coaching

Clinicians who do successfully elicit behavioral rehearsal can still minimize the impact of the rehearsal if they fail to provide needed corrective feedback and coaching. Skills trainers seem as vulnerable to this problem as individual therapists. Some therapists fail to notice relevant errors and omissions, either because they have not learned the skill well enough to identify such issues or because they became unmindful during the session. To address the former reason, therapists might need more basic training about the skill(s) (e.g., reading books, watching videos) or more feedback from the team on session recordings and more role plays with the consultation team. A turn as a skills trainer will also help if the co-trainer does not share the problem. To treat persistent deficits in attention, therapists might need more mindfulness practices related to in-session distractions or better physical care to enhance alertness (e.g., sufficient sleep, exercise prior to sessions, fresh air during sessions). Other therapists notice the errors and omissions but do not correct them, either because they have not learned well enough how to provide feedback or coaching or because cognitions or emotions interfere. Role-playing during consultation meetings on how to give feedback and coaching can effectively address that skills deficit. Cognitions that inhibit giving feedback and coaching include beliefs that clinicians should not invalidate clients, that clients should like them, and that feedback will punish clients who will then avoid further practice. Emotions that inhibit feedback include fears about clients becoming angry and guilt about "pushing" clients. The solutions for any particular therapist depend on the specific thoughts and emotions controlling the therapist's behavior.

While watching a session recording, clinicians on Rita's DBT team observed that her therapist had failed to provide feedback and coaching of Rita's rehearsal of interpersonal effectiveness skills. In particular, the therapist did not shape Rita's voice tone and body posture, both of which conveyed anger. Failure to change these behaviors had decreased the effectiveness of Rita's skills application on the unit. Rita's therapist had noticed the problems with voice tone and posture but fear and associated cognitions had inhibited her from highlighting them. In analyzing her failure to shape Rita's behaviors, Rita's therapist realized that she had made potentially inaccurate assumptions about the behaviors. As Rita had previously refused to role-play at all, the therapist automatically assumed that any corrective feedback would punish Rita's willingness in this session to role-play. The team suggested that the therapist examine the evidence for this assumption by discussing it with Rita. They also suggested ways that the therapist could minimize any punishing consequences and balance them with more reinforcement. The therapist also recognized that she feared that any shaping of the skills would prompt Rita to make further complaints about her. As Rita's past behavior warranted the fear, the team first validated the fear, both verbally and by problem solving how to minimize the likelihood of complaints and to tackle any threats that occurred. The team also helped the therapist to rehearse opposite action, as the fear's intensity had reached unwarranted levels. Finally, the therapist role-played providing effective feedback to Rita about the postural and voice tone problems interwoven with validating the difficulty of the task for Rita and praising her efforts.

Providing Inaccurate or Incomplete Feedback and Coaching

Clinicians who do provide corrective feedback and coaching sometimes provide erroneous or oversimplified feedback and coaching. For example, in some cases when clients have rehearsed mindfully describing their inner state and described an aversion (e.g., "I hate my ex-husband"), their therapists have "corrected" them erroneously by labeling the statement as judgmental. When having clients rehearse pros and cons, some therapists allow clients to simply recite a number of consequences with as little thought or emotion as they would have reading a shopping list. Though accurate, such reciting often minimizes the impact of the skill. The most common reasons for these problems include the same reasons that clinicians provide inaccurate or incomplete information during skills acquisition, namely having insufficient knowledge of the skill(s) and minimizing the complexity of the skill. Fortunately, the same solutions will help. In addition, some clinicians have not developed the ability to coach, regardless of the exact skill. Coaching requires noticing errors and omissions, highlighting them in a way that maintains the client's engagement, providing specific instructions and modeling as in skills acquisition, and finally motivating the client to rehearse the skill again, and perhaps repeating the whole process yet again. Therapists can develop this ability, however, by watching training videos, role playing with the consultation team, and practicing a lot with clients.

SKILLS GENERALIZATION

Conceptualization and Strategies

Skills generalization procedures assist clients in transferring the skills that they have learned in treatment to their daily lives. Clients behave skillfully sometimes but not at other times. Others individuals then accuse clients of "just not wanting" to behave skillfully when the clients do "want" to behave skillfully but have not learned to generalize skills across varying contexts. Two kinds of procedures are used to maximize skills generalization across the various contexts that clients encounter. Stimulus generalization involves identifying opportunities to practice a single skill in a variety of contexts, whereas response generalization involves teaching clients how to choose and combine a variety of skills options for a single context. In addition to ensuring that clients have the capability to implement a range of skills for a range of contexts, therapists must also attend to the contingencies of implementation. Therapists incorporate generalization procedures when they both prepare for and later review clients' skills implementation.

Enhance Stimulus Generalization

To enhance stimulus generalization, therapists identify relevant external and internal contexts and encourage clients to practice skills in these settings. Ideally, these contexts will vary in both cues and contingencies, as both determine how well skills generalize. The skills training manual (Linehan, 1993b, 2014) contains weekly homework assignments for clients to complete and then review the following week. To increase the likelihood that the client can complete the homework with success, skills trainers guide clients toward choosing relatively simply or easy contexts for these assignments. Individual therapists also assign homework, but base the assignments on each client's own skills deficits. Individual therapists might also leave their office to conduct skills strengthening in settings where clients will use the skills. During pretreatment, for example, clients who anticipate that anxiety might inhibit their attendance in skills class often benefit from rehearsing anxiety management skills in their skills classroom rather than in their therapists' office. Skills coaches provide coaching while clients are still in their natural environments.

Relevant external environments for stimulus generalization include both physical environments and interpersonal environments. For example, research has revealed a relationship between heat and aggression (see Anderson, 1989, for a review). Nighttime presents a notably different set of stimuli than daytime. Some clients experience more stress in noisy environments than in quiet ones. With respect to interpersonal contexts, the multimodal nature of DBT immediately provides multiple contexts in which to practice skills. Clients implement skills acquired and strengthened in the skills group with their individual therapist and vice versa. The consultation team agreement referred to as the "consistency agreement" (Linehan, 1993a) explicitly states that unanimity in therapists' responses, methods, or styles of treatment implementation is not required. This agreement functions primarily to enhance generalization. Thus, therapists may use different methods to teach skills, express contrasting levels of irreverence, have variable thresholds for reinforcement, or may require different interpersonal behaviors before providing reinforcement. DBT clinicians can then provide corrective feedback and coaching to clients if needed, thus providing an optimal environment for clients to experiment with implementation. Many DBT clients also have non-DBT treatment networks (e.g., psychiatrist, social worker) that provide additional contexts in which the client can practice skills. Primarily, however, therapists focus on helping clients generalize skills to familial and other social contexts.

While variations in external context provide numerous opportunities for generalization, often the most significant generalization challenge for clients comes from the significant fluctuations in their internal psychological and physiological environments. Skills effective in one internal state can evaporate altogether in another! For example, research on self-control (see Gaillot & Baumeister, 2007, for a review) has demonstrated that lower levels of glucose predict worse executive functioning, emotion regulation, and impulse control. Emotions, mood disorders, auditory hallucinations, and lack of sleep can equally diminish the capacity for skills. To assist clients in transferring skills from in-session strengthening to out-of-session generalization, therapists try to anticipate the internal states in which the client will use the skill and try to incorporate them into the rehearsal. For example, although Rita's anger during her session made it more difficult for the therapist to assist with strengthening Rita's interpersonal skills, the presence of the anger also created a more "realistic" environment. Alternatively, simply asking clients to imagine a specific emotion or other internal state may suffice.

Ensuring that clients remember to practice a skill in all relevant contexts sometimes necessitates that the therapist help the client to create associations between a stimulus in the context and the skill or to add a relevant stimulus to the context. For example, Jane needed to practice mindfulness and urge surfing when dressing. Her therapist suggested that she repeatedly walk to her closet and look at it while thinking about those skills in order to form an association such that seeing the closet would prompt her to practice the skills. Her therapist also suggested that she attach a sign saying "MINDFULNESS" to the door until the association had developed. They later applied a similar set of strategies in the bathroom. Furthermore, Jane's therapist assigned her homework that required her to practice every standard bathroom task mindfully. Susan's therapist held up her finger and uttered a single mindfulness instruction whenever Susan said something unmindful. Though this functioned primarily as skills strengthening, Susan reported that after weeks of this whenever she had certain unmindful thoughts outside of session a memory of the therapist would flash into her mind. Susan's therapist also encouraged her to use notes or signs in critical places, such as on her evening bag.

Enhance Response Generalization

Response generalization addresses the reality that not all skills work across all contexts and that most situations require multiple skills. This reality seems particularly true for clients who have such complex problems that they need a treatment like DBT. Response generalization procedures aim to ensure that clients have a sufficient breadth of skills to respond flexibly in different contexts and that they can combine these options in any given situation. The original skills training manual (Linehan, 1993b), for example, lists 176 options for increasing positive emotions through pleasant events. It identifies several general options for surviving crises, including self-soothing. It then suggests multiple ways to implement self-soothing, as not everyone likes lotion and taking a bubble bath at work would likely cause another crisis. Individual therapists contribute to response generalization when they verify that clients know multiple skills for a single controlling variable. To decrease emotions, for example, clients learn skills to change their physiology, reorient their attention, and act opposite to emotional urges. To decrease physiological arousal for "hot" emotions, Jane learned to immerse her face in cold water (Linehan, 2014), pace her breathing, and relax her muscles. The cold water proved most effective, but applied to few contexts. Clients need skills to help them immediately change aspects of a situation and skills that will help them to prevent the situation from reoccurring. Therapists try to ensure that clients develop different skills for different types of links in the chain, as Jane's and Susan's solutions analyses (see Boxes 4.2 and 4.3, respectively, in Chapter 4) illustrate. Therapists also teach clients the principles that they use to generate solutions for clients, including how to match links with solutions (see Chapter 4) and how to sequence solutions. For example, intense emotions often necessitate changing physiological arousal or reorienting attention to decrease the emotion before clients can use skills requiring more cognitive capacity effectively. Interpersonal success often necessitates implementing "GIVE" skills before "DEAR MAN" skills. Therapists must also guard against clients using only a limited set of skills, particularly crisis survival skills or other short-term solutions, when other skills would be a better match. Over time, therapists and skills coaches alike decrease generating solutions themselves and require more solution generation from the client.

Jane's case provides an example of the complexity of skills often needed to achieve a single goal. When Jane told her therapist that she "felt stressed" by her mother always "watching her" and that it "made her too self-conscious" to try many of her DBT skills, she and her therapist rehearsed using the "DEAR MAN" skills to request time alone for DBT skills practice as the most useful solution. After several sessions, Jane reported that her mother remained as vigilant as ever, had expressed reluctance to give her time alone, and had justified this by saying that Jane's self-harm urges meant that time alone "would not be a good idea." Jane and her therapist invited her mother into the next session to explain the strategy. During this discussion, the therapist requested that Jane practice asking her mother for the time. Though the content of what Jane said indicated some interpersonal skills strength, the manner in which she said it indicated a significant weakness. The therapist noticed that Jane asked in a timid voice, with her head down and slightly turned away. She was breathing faster and appeared highly emotional. When asked, Jane reported feeling embarrassed and fearful. Her mother reported that this behavior had also occurred at home and increased her anxiety about Jane. The therapist first focused on treating Jane's emotions, particularly using paced breathing for the fear, changing body posture for the embarrassment, and increasing voice tone for both. These skills also made Jane appear more interpersonally confident. They also incorporated additional interpersonal skills to validate the mother's anxiety and to negotiate a solution that addressed her concerns. After a couple of role plays with her mother, Jane's skills had improved and her mother agreed to the time alone. Her mother also reported that she herself felt less anxious.

The consequences of using a skill determine whether that skill generalizes nearly as much as the ability to use the skill does. If clients' internal and external environments do not reinforce a skill, the skill will extinguish. Clients frequently live in environments that reinforce maladaptive behaviors and punish skillful behaviors. This applies equally to internal and external environments. For example, most clients easily acquire the skill of self-soothing but using the skill is often punished by their judgmental thoughts, such as "I don't deserve to take care of myself" or "I'm being selfish," and consequent guilt or shame. When Jack started to regulate his emotions better and use more interpersonal skills, some newer non-DBT staff members on the unit expressed concerns that he was hiding something or trying to manipulate them. Jack then resorted to less skillful behavior in the presences of these staff members.

Erroneous expectations about a skill can result in extinction rather than reinforcement of the skill. Though clinicians will have taught clients what to expect during skills acquisitions procedures, clients may still have inaccurate assumptions. Clients may expect that a single skill will suffice when the situation requires several. Some clients anticipate that after only basic skills acquisition and strengthening implementing skills will lead to significant changes in themselves and others in their environment. For example, clients new to the treatment and keen to improve their interpersonal relationships may decide after only a few interpersonal effectiveness classes to tackle major long-term marital difficulties. Though resolving such difficulties will require competence in interpersonal skills, few clients have enough competence early in treatment and such situations require more than just interpersonal skills. Successful planning for generalization and later reviewing implementation often necessitates assessing and moderating clients' expectations about likely outcomes.

Learning new skills inevitably necessitates more work, more risk, or limited reinforcement until clients have developed some proficiency. For example, opposite action can dramatically decrease emotions, but it involves multiple component skills, including correctly identifying the emotion, identifying multiple actions associated with the emotion (including cognitive behaviors), and generating opposite behaviors for each action and then implementing the opposite action. Not surprisingly, clients may not experience extensive changes to their emotions while initially learning the skill. Therefore, clients usually need validation regarding the difficulty of learning and other types of reinforcement from therapists to motivate them through the learning phase. Ironically, limited but reliable success with one skill or skill set can lead to overuse of that skill and decrease the generalization of other skills. This typically arises when the skills group teaches a skill already well established in a client's repertoire or the client learns a new skill that reliably produces immediate results with little effort. Clients' implementation of distraction typifies this pattern, as many clients are highly accomplished at distraction such that they can depend on it to decrease their distress immediately. The problem arises when the distraction becomes so reinforcing that clients have little motivation to implement other skills that require more learning, effort, or patience but will produce better long-term results.

Optimize Consequences of Skill Use

Skills generalization procedures also attempt to optimize the consequences for using skills. Stimulus procedures enable therapists to assess consequences for skills use in a variety of contexts and to identify the most reinforcing environments. For example, Jack and his therapist identified which staff members would reinforce Jack's skillful requests for help with problem solving and which members would likely extinguish the behavior. Response generalization procedures include teaching clients how to adapt or combine their skills to maximize reinforcement and minimize extinction or punishment, as in the example with Jane's mother. In some instances, incorporating a skill that increases attention to the full range of existing contingencies for using other skills increases the likelihood of implementing those skills. For example, Susan had the interpersonal skills to say "No" to the man in the bar, but attended more to the immediate reinforcement for saying "Yes," namely happiness, than to the less immediate negative consequences. She never considered that saying "No" could have its own rewards. To address this imbalance, her therapist helped Susan to review the pros and cons of saying "No" versus "Yes." They attended to immediate (e.g., "Yes" wins happiness), intermediate (e.g., "Yes" leads to shame and guilt), and long-term consequences (e.g., "Yes" risks losing relationship with boyfriend and suicidal urges, "No" achieves goal of stopping promiscuity and may elicit a sense of mastery). This attention to a wider range of consequences immediately shifted Susan's motivation to say "No." To increase the likelihood that Susan would use pros and cons outside of the session, she put the list on her phone to review before visiting bars and even at bars.

Max's case illustrates how therapists encourage skills use across contexts, attend to contingencies, and add both new skills and environments to maximize reinforcement. Although progressing in therapy, Max continued to have substance abuse problems that usually occurred when he saw his friends who used drugs, a number of whom aggressively pushed drugs on him. As Max's interpersonal skills with his therapist and family had improved, his therapist suggested practicing some "DEAR MAN" skills with those friends who pushed drugs. Max emitted a withering look and said that while he would try these "weird" skills with "regular people" like his parents and school teachers, he just did not think that they would work with drug dealers. Rather than dismissing this out of hand, the therapist encouraged Max to role-play a drug-dealing friend while the therapist took the role of Max so that she could learn what he "was up against." Following several explorations of different scenarios, they decided to use some judicious lying about his medication, implying that he did not need to take illegal drugs when his legal ones worked so well. They thought this, along with courtesy, validation, an easy manner, and no apologies might work best. The therapist worked on her skills to impersonate a suspicious, aggressive, drug dealer in order to help Max practice this strategy and was delighted when Max congratulated her on her newly developed skills. Though Max successfully implemented his new interpersonal skills with the friends, he eventually decided that he wanted friends who would reinforce a wider range of skillful behavior, and his therapist then helped him toward this new goal.

Common Problems

Neglecting Generalization

Some therapists scarcely attend to generalization at all, while other therapists attend to some aspects but miss others. These problems can occur if therapists do not know how to apply generalization procedures, but more often occur if therapists believe that generalization will occur through psychological osmosis, that is, automatically without planning or effort. When clients do not use skills outside the session, these therapists tend to assume "He's being willful" or "She doesn't want to change." With some therapists, the problem is quickly solved by cognitive modification in the form of didactic information on generalization and clinical examples of reasons clients do not use skills. Other therapists might need the consultation team to highlight repeated incidents of the assumption for an extended period. Some therapists also need a bit of contingency management in which they learn not only how their assumption is incorrect, but also how it adversely impacts the client's treatment. For example, one inpatient therapist remained attached to the "osmosis" hypothesis until she returned from an extended absence and saw how much more her clients used skills after working with another DBT therapist who attended to generalization.

Not Ensuring That Clients Have a Sufficient Skill Set

Specific aspects of generalization that therapists may miss include ensuring that clients know how to implement a range of skills, teaching clients to recognize when to use which skills, and attending to the consequences of skills implementation. Therapist errors that contribute to clients not having a sufficient range of skills for generalization include not identifying when clients use only a limited range of skills, automatically assuming that clients have implemented skills competently, and not assigning homework for skills that have not generalized. Reviewing the skills side of the diary card for patterns of use offers therapists an efficient way to check for any patterns of limited use. Neglect of an entire skills module, such as emotion regulation skills, appears obvious on the diary card, but other patterns do not. For example, some clients implement skills across the modules but neglect all skills related to taking care of themselves, such as increasing positive emotions, the "PLEASE" skills, self-soothing, and the "FAST" skills. Though therapists also watch for patterns during analyses of target behaviors, consultation teams can detect patterns that a therapist has missed by reviewing each others' written BCAs and solution analyses. Therapists would then assess whether clients' limited skills resulted from a lack of cues to use the skill, a skills deficit, or problematic contingencies.

Failing to assess whether clients have implemented skills competently appears most obvious when a therapist automatically accepts a client's statement that the skill "didn't work." The skill may not work for the client, but an assessment of what the client actually said or did often reveals deficits in the implementation. For example, clients might say that "wise mind" did not work when they used only reasonable mind, or that opposite action for fear did not work when they inhibited urges to flee but maintained catastrophic thinking and tense body posture and facial expression. Listening to recordings during consultation meetings can help to detect whether a therapist has failed to assess a client's competency. The team can also identify reasons for the therapist's error (e.g., does not believe in the efficacy of the skills, little experience of how clients can misunderstand skills, fearful of invalidating the client, not knowing how to assess competency) and then help the therapist generate and implement related solutions.

Some therapists do highlight and correct clients' skills deficits in the session but then fail to give related homework assignments. For example, one therapist complained to the consultation team that every week she noticed the client's judgmental thoughts, both during the session and in the client's chain analyses, and had coached the client on how to apply mindfulness skills, but she not heard any improvement. After listening to part of the therapist's last session, the team commended her on her high competence in applying skills strengthening in the session, but noticed that she had not assigned any mindfulness homework for skills generalization outside of the session.

Not Assisting Clients to Recognize When to Use Which Skills

Therapists sometimes overlook the extent to which generalization involves the ability to recognize when to use which skills, as well as how to use them. With time, effective skills implementation can become automatic, but initially clients will have to choose consciously when and which skills to implement. Therapists' errors include not helping clients to acquire principles of skills selection, not strengthening clients' skills selection capacity, and not helping clients to establish environmental cues for skills use. With regard to the first error, some therapists assume that because they modeled skill selection during weekly solution analyses, their clients must have learned the basic principles. Selecting skills to implement, however, requires recognizing the need for skills; the capacity to identify controlling variables of a problematic affect, cognition, or behavior (including both internal and external cues and contingencies); and finally to select an appropriately matched set of skills from a myriad of skills. Skill selection is thus a highly complex skill itself. Clients often need their individual therapists to provide very specific guidelines and sometimes even written instructions or diagrams. Requesting that clients record links from their chain in one column and corresponding solutions in another may facilitate the creation of problem-skill associations more than just writing a summary list of skills to practice.

Besides not educating clients sufficiently about how to select skills, therapists can fail to shape clients' skills selection capabilities, either by not requiring that clients contribute increasing amounts to solution analyses over time or by not correcting critical errors in their skills selection. For example, many therapists request that their clients complete a written BCA as homework but fail to request a matching solution analysis. When one individual therapist complained that her client still phoned for coaching frequently after many months of treatment, the team role-played a call with the therapist and noticed that she immediately started generating solutions for the client rather than coaching the client on how to identify solutions. Further analysis revealed that the combination of the client's distress and lack of time for coaching made the therapist so anxious that she wanted to identify as many solutions as quickly as possible. The team suggested that the therapist require the client to have generated an increasing number of relevant skills before phoning the therapist and that the therapist use the phone consultation to coach the client to select skills if the client had missed critical ones. Another individual therapist did ask his client to generate solutions for the unwarranted fear that had elicited her suicidal urges. The client generated and implemented several skills, but later reported that although the fear initially decreased, it soon returned and she became exhausted trying to persist with the skills. When the therapist reviewed the client's solution implementation with the team, they noticed that the client had generated only distress tolerance skills and had missed the emotion regulation and mindfulness skills that could produce long-lasting effects. In a third case, the therapist of a forensic client noticed several months into treatment that the client still used only distraction to decrease warranted guilt of moderate strength rather than repair, but the therapist had not confronted this pattern because she feared that the client would become angry with her for challenging his skills selection. To minimize the likelihood of the client becoming angry, the team role-played with the therapist how to orient to and conduct the implementation review in a style that communicated and cultivated curiosity rather confrontation.

Reasons for not helping clients to establish environmental cues include failing to recognize the need, not knowing how to create stimulus–response associations, and assuming that a client's lack of skills implementation results from willfulness or "commitment problems." For example, during a session the therapist and client reviewed the pros and cons of overdosing. At the next session, the client reported that she had overdosed and revealed that she had not used pros and cons because she could not remember them, so her therapist requested that the client write a list as they reviewed them. After learning the following week that the client still had not used pros and cons to try to prevent an overdose, the therapist concluded that the client "just did not want to change." When she sought consultation from the team, they noted, in part, that the list may remind her client of how to implement the pros and cons but not remind her when she needed to implement the skill. Moving the list from the client's rather chaotic DBT folder to the cabinet where she kept her medication significantly increased her use of the skill.

Not Attending to Consequences of Skills Use

Finally, therapists can fail to attend to and adjust how consequences reinforce, extinguish, or punish skills implementation. For example, Rita's complaint about her therapist always focusing on skills and not understanding her resulted partly from the therapist having previously failed to attend to the contingencies for skills use. In particular, prior to the solution analysis presented in Chapter 4 (see Box 4.1), Rita's therapist had pushed Rita to use opposite action for anger. After trying it on the unit, Rita reported that the skill "didn't work" and that she "still felt awful." After assessing specifically how Rita had used the skill, the therapist concluded that Rita had implemented the skill correctly and that Rita simply "didn't want to get better." The therapist discussed this problem with team members, and they asked what else happened after Rita used the skill. When the therapist assessed the consequences with Rita, she discovered that the skill had successfully reduced the anger but then Rita began to experience anxiety, as the anger had functioned to distract her from the anxiety. The therapist then addressed the problematic contingencies. Chapter 8 discusses contingency management in more detail.

CHAPTER 6

STIMULUS CONTROL AND EXPOSURE

Although skills deficits increase the likelihood that clients will use target behaviors to solve problems, motivational variables also control the probability of those behaviors. On the antecedent side, a prompting event or other stimulus can directly elicit a maladaptive impulse. For example, the sight of alcohol bottles can directly elicit an urge to drink alcohol. At other times, a stimulus elicits an emotional response that then motivates maladaptive behavior or inhibits adaptive behavior. For example, social situations can elicit fear that then motivates bingeing on alcohol or inhibits conversing with other people. Stimulus control problems also occur when a stimulus fails to motivate a normative behavior or to inhibit a maladaptive behavior. For many clients with sleeping disorders, the sensations of lying on a bed in the dark fail to cue a normal "sleepy" response. In some situations, the stimulus itself is problematic such as a former abuser arriving at a client's home. In other situations, the response elicited by the stimulus is the problem. For one client with binge eating as a target, seeing any television program elicited eating impulses because she ate so often while watching television. In another case, a client became intensely fearful whenever anyone rang the doorbell; she would hide in her bedroom rather than look through the peephole, even if she expected a friend or her social worker. Many BCAs reveal that both the stimulus and the response warrant change, and they identify a pattern of escalating, dysfunctional stimulus–response relationships. This chapter focuses on the treatment of problematic stimuli and problematic emotional and overt behavioral responses to stimuli. Because of the biosocial theory's emphasis on emotion as a motivating variable, the chapter particularly attends to this type of stimulus–response relationship.

Stimulus–response relationships can be biologically hardwired but are more likely conditioned. Through the process of classical conditioning, any stimulus can begin to elicit problematic responses, but similar stimulus–response patterns occur for most clients. Although the types of external stimuli outnumber the types of internal stimuli, internal stimuli can prove equally motivating or inhibiting. External stimuli controlling DBT targets include the sight of medication eliciting an urge to overdose, the smell of food eliciting an urge to binge, and the sound of an alarm clock leading to a depressed mood. Many anxiety disorders involve external stimuli, such as the outdoors, crowds, animals, airplanes aloft, and social situations. Interpersonal stimuli can also elicit direct emotional or overt behavioral responses. For example, Rita's BCA suggests that she responded with anxiety to her psychiatrist's inquiry even before she interpreted the inquiry. Internal stimuli controlling DBT targets include somatic sensations leading to panic and "feeling full" leading to vomiting. Collectively, these stimuli elicit the full range of basic emotional responses. For one client, the sight of his girlfriend talking with her male colleagues consistently prompted unwarranted jealousy that led to violent impulses. In Susan's case, subsequent BCAs revealed that the stimulus of a man smiling at her frequently led to promiscuous sexual behavior because it elicited happiness that then prompted an urge to flirt, which led to sexual invitations. These stimuli and emotions then lead, directly or indirectly, to the full range of target behaviors.

DBT therapists and clients have two main chances for changing stimulus–response relationships that lead to dysfunctional behavior; they can apply solutions either to the stimulus or to the response. This chapter discusses CBT principles and procedures involved in changing both sides of the stimulus–response relationship, focusing particularly on stimulus control and exposure procedures. Several factors determine whether the solution analysis focuses on changing the stimulus or the response or includes solutions for both. Therapists consider which element of the relationship is most unjustified, abnormal, or otherwise problematic. For example, in the case of the client who became intensely fearful and hid at the sound of the doorbell, the stimulus did not warrant such an intense fear response. Thus, the therapist focused on changing the response with exposure. In some cases, both the stimulus and response warrant change. For example, Carmella, a client with severe acne, had extreme shame responses to her acne and its scars that led her to miss therapy appointments and avoid employment. She and her therapist combined stimulus control, in the form of medication and makeup, to minimize the appearance of blemishes and exposure to reduce the intensity of the shame about the remaining blemishes. Therapists and clients also consider how easily clients can implement the solutions. For example, one client who was being harassed, primarily via phone calls, stopped the harassment but still experienced extreme fear when the phone rang, despite having changed her phone number. An analysis indicated that during the period of the harassment she had become classically conditioned to the ring tone on her phone. Although the ring tone no longer warranted the fear response, the client chose to change the tone rather than use exposure because the former required little effort or time and proved very effective. Therapists must also attend to how well the solution will generalize. For example, if the harassed client had previously had a popular ring tone, changing the tone on her phone might have proved ineffective because she would have heard it on other phones and still respond with fear. Initial solution analyses sometimes emphasize easier solutions in the short term, while developing longer-term solutions that require more time and effort to implement.

STIMULUS CONTROL

Conceptualization and Strategies

Stimulus control refers to changing stimuli either to reduce maladaptive behaviors or to increase skillful behaviors. Clients can often directly change a stimulus. For situations in which a stimulus contributes to motivating maladaptive behavior or inhibiting adaptive behavior, clients can remove or avoid the stimulus or decrease its intensity, duration, or frequency. Alternatively, clients might increase a stimulus for situations in which it consistently fails to elicit a normative, adaptive response. Clients can also introduce new stimuli to inhibit maladaptive behaviors or to prompt adaptive behavior. Clients can also control the motivational aspect of the stimulus by modifying their experience of it. They can change either their attention to the stimulus or the meaning or value they ascribe to the stimulus. Behavioral treatments have developed multiple stimulus control techniques over time. The use of the techniques varies across treatments, and the techniques sometimes overlap. This section, therefore, focuses on general strategies and principles rather than specific techniques.

   As with the choice of stimulus control versus exposure, the selection of stimulus control strategies depends on the conceptual match between the link and the solution, the ease of altering the stimuli, whether the alteration generalizes to relevant contexts and, of course, the overall effectiveness of the solution. In many instances, clients can combine stimulus control strategies. Carmella's case demonstrates several of these points. Her acne and associated scars were minor, but sufficiently noticeable to have caused comments in some social situations, so the stimulus did warrant attention. Her insurance company designated the acne as a medical condition and the scars as cosmetic, so Carmella could afford new medications to remove the acne but not an effective treatment to remove the scars. Although the medications successfully reduced the intensity and duration of the acne, they did not remove it entirely. To minimize the appearance of the remaining acne and the scars, Carmella found a particular cosmetic and learned special application tips. As described in further detail below, her therapist also coached her on how to alter her attention to both the acne and the scars.

Change Stimuli

DECREASE PROBLEMATIC STIMULI

Removing or avoiding a stimulus generally works best when it is inherently unhealthy or the client has the capacity to remove or avoid it across relevant contexts without causing other problems. Physical abuse perhaps provides the most obvious type of inherently unhealthy stimulus requiring removal. For stimuli that cause problems only because of conditioning, therapists and clients can consider removal or avoidance if it seems easily implemented and either generalizes well or helps in the short term while long-term solutions are implemented. When clients cannot or reasonably do not want to completely remove or avoid a stimulus, they still can consider decreasing the intensity, duration, or frequency of the stimulus. For example, in response to invalidating communications by family members, many clients experience warranted negative emotions that then lead to urges to engage in a variety of target behaviors. Some clients have decided to disrupt such chains by having no contact with those family members because the relationship provides no benefit. Other clients learn that the negative communications happen only in certain contexts, so they decide to avoid those contexts. One client noticed that her mother judged and ridiculed her only when drunk, so the client avoided phoning her mother during her mother's preferred drinking times. Many clients cannot avoid the aversive interpersonal stimulus without avoiding the individual, but they do not want to sever the relationship because it also provides useful benefits. Modifying the intensity, duration, or frequency of the stimulus may prove more useful in such cases. Briefer time periods with these individuals effectively prevents emotions from becoming overwhelming for many clients. One client learned that spending time with her parents separately rather than together effectively reduced the intensity and frequency of invalidating comments.

Planning the removal or avoidance of a cue involves an assessment of whether a cue causes problems only in certain contexts or regardless of the wider context. The more varied the contexts, the more the therapy will need to attend to generalization. For Scott, an adult outpatient, seeing alcohol or alcohol-related advertisements in bars consistently elicited impulsive drinking, whereas seeing such cues at home or at the supermarket elicited urges only if he already had moderately strong emotions. Restaurants, however, did not elicit impulsive drinking urges at all. Scott committed to remove all alcohol from his home permanently so that it would not prompt drinking during unpredictable periods of emotional vulnerability. He also agreed to avoid the alcohol aisle at the grocery store regardless of his emotional state, because doing so made it easier to implement the solution. For social reasons, Scott did not want to avoid bars, so he and his therapist agreed to a temporary avoidance of this stimulus until Scott had strengthened his skills and developed other solutions to reduce or inhibit urges to drink in that context. They could not, however, remove or even reduce advertisements for alcohol, as these usually occurred in environments that Scott could not control, such as television commercials during programs that Scott really enjoyed.

For Jane, television programs and other media about women's bodies or weight could elicit anxiety, envy, or shame whenever she viewed them, though, like many clients with eating disorders, she often sought these stimuli. The sight or feel of various body parts and the sensations associated with several pieces of clothing could elicit moderate fear, queasiness, or shame, though the jeans elicited these responses more consistently than any other clothing. Only toilets that Jane had used previously for vomiting elicited an impulse to vomit, and they elicited the impulse only if Jane already had queasiness or urges to vomit. During their initial solution analysis of vomiting, Jane's therapist suggested not watching dieting programs, because the program appeared to prompt the entire chain and Jane could easily remove the stimulus. Although Jane could not avoid all media about women's bodies or dieting, subsequent solution analyses led her to remove all of the dieting media that she had collected. Jane also made a long-term commitment not to seek information about how to engage in eating-disordered behavior and a short-term commitment not to seek television programming or other media on other relevant topics until she had learned skills to manage the emotions that these media elicited. This solution proved difficult to implement, as her current emotional state significantly influenced her motivation to implement the solution. In the initial analysis, Jane's therapist suggested that Jane surf the urge to try on the jeans, but as with avoiding media, motivational factors decreased the likelihood of Jane implementing urge surfing. Therefore, during a subsequent analysis in which the jeans played a role, Jane's therapist suggested that Jane temporarily remove the jeans from her closet, and Jane complied. Because the fit of the clothing did not warrant the intensity of the emotions that it elicited, nor could Jane practically remove all of her clothing, she and her therapist eventually applied exposure procedures to treat the dysfunctional stimulus–response relationship. In the initial solution analysis for vomiting, Jane's therapist had already suggested walking away from the bathroom as a solution for the urge to vomit. To the extent that Jane implemented this solution, the solution also effectively removed the cue for spontaneous vomiting.

Decreasing problematic stimuli often requires other solutions to directly modify a stimulus or to remove obstacles to implementation. For example, as mentioned in Chapter 5, removing the man from her home required that Susan use interpersonal skills. Scott needed a range of solutions to avoid entering bars. The solutions included focusing on effectiveness and reviewing aversive consequences when friends invited him to "go out drinking" and using interpersonal skills to persuade friends to meet him at other places. If friends teased him about not drinking or not visiting bars, he needed a combination of mindfulness, cognitive restructuring, opposite action, and interpersonal effectiveness. Initially, Scott did not believe that he could successfully avoid visiting bars, but with in-session rehearsal during several analyses he developed the required capacity and some particularly impressive interpersonal skills. Despite the number of additional solutions required for success, he could more easily avoid the stimulus of a bar early in treatment than inhibit urges to drink in a bar.

INCREASE USEFUL STIMULI

When a stimulus fails to elicit a normative, adaptive response, the stimulus control may involve increasing the intensity, frequency, or duration of the stimuli. For example, the BCA for one client revealed that she had arrived very late to her morning skills training group partly because she had not awoken when her alarm sounded. Having established that this occurred frequently, the therapist suggested the addition of a loud alarm or two to increase the intensity of the sound. The BCA of the next late arrival to group revealed that adding a loud alarm had awoken the client, but that she had reached out of bed, silenced them, and returned to sleep. This time, the therapist suggested moving the alarms away from the bed so that the client could not remove the stimuli so easily and adding a third alarm, also placed away from the bed but set for a slightly later time in case the client silenced the first two. After the client implemented these solutions, the frequency of late arrivals decreased notably.

Stimulus control can also include the introduction of a new stimulus to prompt effective behavior or to inhibit maladaptive behavior. In many DBT skills training groups, for example, one of the skills trainers phones clients who have not arrived on time to prompt them to attend group. (The solution often has a contingency management effect as well.) Individual therapists may do this for individual sessions if the solution analysis has indicated that such a prompt would help. This solution will not generalize beyond the therapeutic context, but therapists usually need to prioritize immediate session attendance above future generalization. Therapists and clients have created a wide variety of cues to prompt clients to use skills. For example, some clients have programmed their computers to flash messages with skills prompts. Many DBT inpatient units have used their physical space to prompt clients to use skills by placing posters about skills around the unit. Such prompting, however, requires attention to the fact that humans habituate to constant, static prompts relatively quickly. One unit attended to this issue by placing posters with amusing depictions of different skills on the inside of a few bathroom stall doors and then changing the selected posters and doors frequently. This combination of a captive audience and frequent change worked well. The addition of certain stimuli can also increase the motivation to inhibit maladaptive impulses. For example, like many clients, Susan developed a list of negative consequences for overdosing that she kept with her medication as a prompt to consider reasons not to overdose when she had urges.

Change the Experiencing of Stimuli

Without altering a stimulus itself, clients may modify how a stimulus motivates their behavior by changing how they experience or perceive the stimulus. This section describes two main ways of achieving this change. The first focuses on controlling attention to the stimulus. The second focuses on altering the appraisal of the stimulus or associations to it. Though one could argue that these strategies change the response to the stimulus rather than control the stimulus, many of the specific techniques have traditionally appeared among stimulus control procedures, so this chapter has included the strategies in this section.

CONTROL ATTENTION TO STIMULI

The degree to which a stimulus elicits a response appears to depend largely on the degree of attention paid to the stimulus. Research has well established that the amount of attention paid to physically painful stimuli significantly predicts the amount of pain reported (e.g., Bantick et al., 2002; Longe et al., 2001; Rode, Salkovskis, & Jack, 2001). Subsequent research has focused on how attention controls painful emotions as well. This research (e.g., McRae et al., 2010; Sheppes & Meiran, 2007; Thiruchselvam, Blechert, Sheppes, Rydstrom, & Gross, 2011) initially demonstrated that directing attention away from affectively salient aspects of a situation reduced both the subjective intensity of emotions and activity in affective areas of the brain. More recent research (Thiruchselvam, Hajcak, & Gross, 2012) has indicated that even after a negative emotional stimuli has entered working memory, selectively attending to neutral versus arousing aspects of the stimuli still mediated both the subjective experience and related neural activity. Thus, attention to a stimulus can elicit stronger emotional responses and increase the motivation for maladaptive behavior or the inhibition of adaptive behavior. In contrast, an absence of attention to existing, relevant stimuli can result in a lack of motivation for skillful behavior or inhibition of dysfunctional behavior.

Exacerbating the impact of emotional stimuli, individuals may have attentional biases toward stimuli generally associated with negative emotions. In clinical and nonclinical populations alike, anxious individuals particularly have demonstrated an attentional bias toward threat cues (see Bar-Haim, Lamy, Pergamin, Bakermans-Kranenburg, & van Ijzendoorn, 2007, for a meta-analysis; Fox, Mathews, Calder, & Yiend, 2007). More generally, individuals may overly attend to a particular emotional stimulus or emotional aspect of a stimulus and fail to attend to other relevant stimuli or aspects. Essentially, they fail to put a stimulus into its proper perspective. For example, when Carmella, the client with acne, looked into a mirror, she focused on her blemishes, sometimes with the aid of a magnifying mirror, and virtually ignored the other aspects of her face. Viewing her face as only a series of blemishes further exacerbated the shame that she felt about the blemishes.

Linehan (1993b) has highlighted the lack of controlled attention among clients with BPD. Therapists can help clients learn to control attention by teaching them how to attend to the actual stimulus in a context, how to discriminate among and contextualize stimuli, and how to focus attention effectively. With her therapist's help, Carmella learned to control her attention to her blemishes in several ways. To correct the contextual bias of her attention, Carmella stopped looking in magnifying mirrors, except when required by a makeup technique. She also learned to evaluate her appearance from the perspective of other people looking at her (e.g., from a few feet away, as having a whole body) rather than from close-ups in the mirror of her face only. As a result of this, she actually discovered that she liked as many aspects of her body as she disliked. Furthermore, Carmella's therapist coached her on how to mindfully attend to tasks that involved looking at or touching her face. In particular, they practiced how she could apply her makeup mindfully by focusing only on that task and returning her attention to the task whenever she became distracted by other stimuli, such as other blemishes. Described by Kabat-Zinn (1994, p. 4) as meaning "paying attention in a particular way: on purpose, in the present moment and non-judgmentally," mindfulness plays the leading role in DBT as the discipline through which clients learn to control their attention. In a recent trial (Soler et al., 2011) investigating the impact of the DBT mindfulness module on attention among clients with BPD, those who received mindfulness training in addition to general psychiatric management (GPM) performed significantly better on a neuropsychology assessment of attention when compared to clients with BPD who received GPM only.

Some clients need additional coaching or training to learn to differentiate between stimuli and to emit a specific behavior in the presence of some stimuli but not in the presence of others. Though a few clients may require formal discrimination training procedures, many clients can learn to attend to the relevant stimuli with simple coaching and without structured trials. For example, Herman, an outpatient, tried to answer every question from the skills trainer in groups to such an extent that it disrupted group. Similarly, whenever his therapist or a skills trainer passed him in the hallway and casually asked, "How are you?" he would respond with a review of all of his problems. These behaviors also caused significant problems with his colleagues at work. When Herman's therapist targeted the group behavior, she first learned that Herman had no awareness of the problem. A BCA then revealed that Herman focused almost exclusively on the question asked by the skills trainers and failed to attend to other relevant cues in the context, namely, other group members. As part of the solution analysis, his therapist helped him to identify other contextual stimuli that warranted attention, particularly the presence of other members trying to speak and skills trainers looking at other group members. A brief assessment of the behavior in the hallway revealed that Herman again attended only to the question and failed to attend to cues that would inhibit a lengthy disclosure of personal problems. His therapist now decided to teach Herman more general principles about how to discriminate among contexts that might elicit an urge to disclose (e.g., public vs. private space, cues related to amount of time available, type of relationship). Though Herman struggled to apply such principles, they did increase his attention to relevant stimuli and helped to inhibit ineffective interpersonal behaviors.

MODIFY ASSOCIATIONS TO STIMULI

Although attention significantly controls responses to stimuli, most responses also depend on conditioning. Therapists may help clients to change their perception or experience of stimuli by helping them to weaken dysfunctional associations, to strengthen functional associations, and to create new functional associations. For example, many clients suffer from insomnia, which can appear either as a target itself or as a link leading to another target. Analyses of insomnia frequently reveal that the common association between bed and sleep has weakened because clients have used their bed extensively for other activities. Reviews of psychological treatments for common types of insomnia (Morin et al., 1999, 2006) have consistently highlighted the efficacy of stimulus control protocols. The protocol for one client particularly emphasized strengthening the bed as a cue for sleeping by restricting the use of the bed to nighttime only and to the function of sleep and sex only. Most importantly, because the stimulus value of the bed had become distorted by the client's prolonged hours of ruminating in bed, the protocol required the client to leave the bed anytime she was continuing to ruminate for more than a few minutes. In another case, a client received a gift from someone who had betrayed her. She liked the gift itself, but whenever she saw it, it elicited anger that then motivated binge eating or drinking. She rejected the idea of disposing of the gift because of its functional and monetary value, adding that a friend had even commented on it favorably a few times. The therapist then suggested giving the gift to the friend, primarily with the aim of reducing the frequency of the cue. When the client implemented the solution, however, her friend received the gift with so much appreciation that the client's experience of the gift completely altered. Whenever she subsequently saw the gift, it elicited happiness instead of anger.

Although the above examples involve a traditional approach to stimulus control, therapists often use other solutions that may achieve the same effect. In particular, cognitive restructuring and mindfulness modify associations by teaching clients a new way to think about an old stimulus. For example, Jamieson, Mendes, and Nock (2013) reported that participants in a reappraisal condition who received information and instructions regarding the utility of acute stress responses had significantly less vasoconstriction and vigilance for threat cues during a stressful task compared with participants who received either no instructions or instructions to ignore the threat source. Mindfulness might teach a client with auditory hallucinations to describe the actual phenomenon without adding any interpretations. Clients might learn to describe the phenomenon as "I'm experiencing hallucinations" or "I'm having the thought that voices are telling me to hurt myself, but it's my brain interpreting the sound as a voice," rather than reifying their thoughts and saying, "The voices are telling me to hurt myself." This solution does not decrease the frequency of auditory hallucinations, but it can effectively change the way that a client responds to the stimulus.

Common Problems

Neglecting Stimulus Control

One of the most notable problems with stimulus control is failing to include it in the solution analysis when appropriate. Consultation teams can detect the absence of potentially effective stimulus control strategies during the review of solution analyses and then analyze the reason for the absence. Frequently, therapists do not even think about stimulus control because they did not learn it during their basic psychotherapy training and Linehan (1993a) does not discuss it in her original treatment manual. In these cases, the consultation team can assign readings, provide clinical examples, and conduct role plays to teach therapists how to conceptualize and implement the various techniques. At other times, therapists use other forms of stimulus control but omit removing or avoiding the stimulus because they have become conditioned themselves to thinking automatically of "avoidance" as "bad." Usually, simply identifying this pattern will prevent therapists from avoiding avoidance, though the consultation team may decide to monitor the therapist's solution analyses for stimulus control or to assign some stimulus control practice to strengthen an association between "avoidance" and "useful."

Failing to Address Obstacles to Implementation

As with other solutions, how therapists respond to clients' evaluation and implementation of stimulus control can create or exacerbate problems. In contrast to most solutions, therapists need to guard against clients or themselves relying exclusively on avoiding or minimizing stimuli when exposure could achieve better results. The section below on exposure discusses this problem in greater detail. Other problems include therapists reinforcing invalid rejections of stimulus control, invalidating valid objections, or failing to treat obstacles to implementation. Susan's therapist struggled with these issues when she and Susan considered stimulus control to decrease the promiscuity. Susan immediately rejected a suggestion to avoid public gathering places if she felt particularly vulnerable to sex with strangers. Her therapist then doubted Susan's commitment to stopping the promiscuity and almost challenged her directly about this. Instead, the therapist assessed the reasons for the rejection and discovered that Susan anticipated that her friends would go without her and that if she stayed home alone, she would ruminate and become more emotional and suicidal. Knowing the accuracy of the latter expectation, her therapist asked Susan to test the accuracy of the former as a homework assignment. They then considered whether the addition of a stimulus in public places would inhibit Susan's urge to flirt. Susan identified that some friends prompted inhibition more than others, but she disliked it when they inhibited her and consequently avoided them sometimes, so she rejected this solution. The therapist now thought that Susan seemed "a bit willful," but she felt "too tired" to challenge Susan or to pursue stimulus control. Noticing that she had become rather unmindful, the therapist refocused her attention on the tasks of solution evaluation. The assessment of what happened when Susan's friends warned her about her behavior revealed that her happiness plummeted and either sadness or anger increased. Susan's therapist then realized that they first needed to address these obstacles before Susan would willingly use stimulus control.

EXPOSURE

Conceptualization and Strategies

DBT therapists employ cue-exposure response prevention procedures when a stimulus repeatedly elicits an emotion due to dysfunctional conditioning and the emotion then motivates maladaptive behaviors. Exposure therapies have demonstrated efficacy for several disorders targeted in DBT, including PTSD (Foa, Hembree, & Rothbaum, 2007), obsessive–compulsive disorder (Foa, Yadin, & Lichner, 2012), and other anxiety disorders (e.g., Abramowitz, Deacon, & Whiteside, 2010; Barlow, 2002). If the therapy has progressed sufficiently to focus specifically on treating one of these disorders, the therapist might apply a course of exposure as the primary solution, following the relevant protocol. Recently, an integration of standard DBT and Foa's prolonged exposure for PTSD (Foa et al., 2007) demonstrated better PTSD-related outcomes when compared to standard DBT in a randomized controlled trial (RCT; Harned, Korslund, & Linehan, 2014). This section reviews the basic principles and practices of exposure and highlights the distinctive features of its application in DBT.

Distinctive DBT Features

In contrast to traditional exposure therapies, which have focused on treating fear responses, DBT therapists apply exposure procedures to a range of unwarranted emotions that control target behaviors. Box 6.1 summarizes several scenarios in which therapists have used exposure to treat emotional responses other than fear. Carmella's therapist, for example, used exposure to treat the unwarranted intensity of Carmella's shame about her acne that led to her missing group sessions and work

Box 6.1. Exposure Scenarios		
Present cue	**Elicit emotion**	**Block behavior**
Acne and associated scars.	Shame	Miss group sessions or work days.
Sensations of fear.	Shame	Hide fear from others, binge drink.
Sensations of shame.	Anger	Swear at teachers.
Therapist announces a scheduled trip.	Sadness	Phone the therapist frequently; beg the therapist not to leave; sob.
Therapist blocks the client's diversions.	Anger	Yell at the therapist; threaten to complain to the manager.

days. Zelda, an outpatient, had a pattern of becoming jealous to an unjustified extent if she saw, or at least suspected, her husband of flirting with other women. When the unjustified jealousy became a variable that contributed to overdosing, Zelda's therapist decided to include exposure as a solution. To test exposure-based procedures to treat other emotions, a pilot study by Rizvi and Linehan (2005), using a single-subject design, investigated the efficacy of exposure-based procedures on dysfunctional shame responses in clients who met criteria for BPD and engaged in suicidal behavior. The results revealed a significant decrease in the average intensity of shame experienced across clients between pretreatment and posttreatment. Though the authors acknowledge the need for a larger, controlled trial, the results of this pilot support extending the use of exposure to the treatment of shame. Also of note, a recently published study of individuals diagnosed with prolonged grief disorder (Bryant et al., 2014) reported that those individuals receiving individual exposure treatment combined with CBT group therapy had significantly greater reductions in prolonged grief and depression compared with those receiving CBT group therapy only.

In some situations the sensations associated with one emotion elicit a conditioned, dysfunctional, second emotion. For example, some clients experience unjustified fear or guilt in response to joy. One patient in a residential treatment center responded with shame any time she experienced fear, because her family had taught her that fear indicated inherent weakness. She would then hide her fear, which meant that she did not receive any help with problem-solving situations that warranted fear. She also frequently became drunk to escape from both emotions. Jamie, an adolescent client, frequently became angry when teachers challenged her disruptive behaviors during class (e.g., talking, giggling, passing notes). She would then swear at the teachers. An analysis of this response revealed warranted shame as a controlling link between the teacher's challenge and the anger. In each of these cases, the therapist used exposure to treat the unwarranted emotion and its related behaviors.

DBT also differs from traditional exposure therapies in the frequency with which therapists use exposure to treat TIBs. As mentioned in Chapter 2, Susan's therapist used exposure to treat Susan's avoidance of the diary card, which initially elicited shame. In the case of Dolores, an adolescent outpatient, whenever her therapist announced an impending trip, Dolores experienced overwhelming sadness. The sadness then motivated sobbing in the session and frequent phone calls to the therapist between sessions. Jack (the patient on a secure unit introduced in Chapter 4), often became very angry when his therapist blocked his attempts to divert away from the target hierarchy, session agenda, or BCA. Jack would then yell at his therapist, threaten to file a complaint about the therapist, or both. In these cases, the therapist used exposure to treat the unwarranted emotion and corresponding TIBs.

Finally, in contrast to the formal structure of standard exposure treatment, exposure in DBT frequently involves interweaving exposure as a solution to treat a link in a specific behavior chain rather than establishing an exposure hierarchy to treat dysfunctional emotional responses to different cues. For example, when Susan's therapist used exposure as a solution for Susan's diary card noncompliance, she limited the application of exposure to the shame elicited by the diary card, either in the session or at home. She did not develop a hierarchy of other cues related to Susan's sexual behavior that elicited an unwarranted degree of shame.

Because DBT includes exposure as a solution for a wider array of emotions leading to a wider array of target behaviors compared with traditional exposure therapies, the solution analysis requires vigilance to ensure exposure is used for unwarranted, rather than warranted, emotional links. For example, the psychiatrist's question at the beginning of Rita's session did not warrant her anxiety, as the psychiatrist did not think that Rita's condition had worsened or that she did not belong on the unit, nor did he pose any other threat. Similarly, the fit of Jane's jeans did not warrant anxiety as a response, particularly given her body mass index (BMI) of 17. Many stimuli, however, warrant the emotion but not the intensity experienced by the client. Though the severity of Carmella's acne and scars did warrant some shame, as demonstrated by others commenting negatively about it, when covered with makeup the acne and scars did not warrant the extreme shame that lead Carmella to avoid her skills training group and employment. Carmella's therapist therefore developed a dialectical solution analysis that included both stimulus control and exposure. In some cases, a stimulus warranted a particular emotional response when the client first entered treatment but no longer warrants the same response because of progress that the client has made during treatment. For example, Chris, an inpatient in a high-security hospital, had a history of physically assaulting others when he became angry. These assaults had resulted in a prison sentence and transfer to the secure hospital for an indefinite stay. When beginning DBT he reported experiencing fear in response to his own anger. This fear motivated him to leave sessions early if he became angry. The consequences of his anger and the fact that he had not yet learned any skills to control his anger justified his fear response. Initially, the therapy heavily targeted assaulting others and treated anger as a controlling variable. Over time, Chris learned various new solutions to manage his anger, stopped his violent behavior, and lowered his violent urges to negligible levels. Unfortunately, he continued to respond with fear to even moderate levels of warranted anger. The fear motivated him to avoid the anger by avoiding situations with any existing or potential interpersonal conflict. If he began to feel even moderate anger toward the therapist during a session, he still would leave the session prematurely, even if the therapist's behavior had warranted the anger. At that point in treatment, the therapist decided to use exposure to treat the fear and leaving the session early.

Standard CBT Procedures

Regardless of the specific context or emotion requiring exposure, DBT therapists apply the standard procedures of exposure treatments and teach clients to apply them. A detailed description of these procedures is beyond the scope of this book, as entire books have been devoted to exposure procedures (e.g., Abramowitz et al., 2010), with some books focusing on using the procedures for a single disorder (e.g., Foa et al., 2007, 2012). Exposure, however, shares with other CBT solutions several of the conceptual and strategic points discussed in Chapter 4 on solution analysis, including conceptually matching solutions with specific links and providing orientation to the procedure. For example, before suggesting exposure, therapists need to ensure that the existing stimulus–response relationship is based on faulty conditioning rather than facts and will not be reinforced during exposure. When orienting to exposure, therapists particularly need to prepare clients for an increase in emotional intensity during the process.

This section focuses on reviewing key principles and strategies particular to the implementation of exposure and provides examples of their application in DBT. Essential to successful implementation, the therapist or client must present the cue that elicits the emotion, and the client must experience the subsequent emotion as it rises and falls. Equally essential to success, the therapist and client must prevent any maladaptive overt or covert action tendencies associated with the emotion. The success of exposure relies both on clearly identifying the cue, the emotion, and the behavior, and then ensuring that the client experiences the cue and the emotion and blocks the behavior.

In Zelda's case, the cue was seeing her husband talking with other women, and the emotion was jealousy. Besides overdosing later, Zelda's immediate behaviors included watching her husband closely, moving closer to him to eavesdrop on his conversation, joining the conversation and demeaning the other woman, steering her husband away from the conversation, or demanding that he leave with her. Exposure required that Zelda tolerate her husband talking to other women without approaching him or even watching him closely during the conversation. She also had to block saying demeaning things about the women or asking her husband to leave after finishing the conversation.

In Chris's case, the cue was the experience of anger, specifically the physical tensing of the muscles, a "sense" of anger, and negative judgments of the therapist. The emotion was fear. Besides leaving the session, maladaptive behaviors included "pushing away" the judgments and inhibiting appropriate expressions of frustration with the therapist. The therapist first taught Chris to implement imaginary exposure, using the last episode of leaving as the imaginary scene. She helped Chris to focus his attention on experiencing the sensations associated with his anger in that scene and to maintain this attention, without escalating or avoiding the sensations, until the fear itself peaked and declined. Chris also practiced allowing his judgmental thoughts rather than preventing them. During this process, the therapist had Chris imagine blocking his avoidant behaviors, namely, leaving the session and inhibiting his expression of frustration with her. After this initial use of exposure, the therapist implemented in vivo exposure whenever Chris became frightened by his own anger during a session.

Presenting the cue properly, either in vivo or with imagery, requires that the therapist and client first specify the relevant cue by identifying its components and contexts. When Jane and her therapist decided to use exposure to treat Jane's unwarranted fear response to the sensations of tight or nonfitting clothing, they discovered that Jane experienced the fear only when she could not fit into the clothing or it felt tight because of the "fatty" parts of her body (e.g., upper arms, belly, or thighs), but not when it did not fit or felt tight because of the "bony" parts (e.g., elbows, wrists, hips). Jane had the same experience regardless of whether she tried the clothing at home or elsewhere, so her therapist asked her to bring a piece to a therapy session so that Jane could receive in vivo coaching during her first exposure trial. After that, Jane practiced daily at home and in store dressing rooms when the opportunity arose.

Rita and her therapist specified the cue that elicited Rita's initial anxiety in the chain as "being asked by a mental health professional 'with authority' about treatment progress in a 'serious' voice tone and without a smile during a session." An "authority" speaking in a "serious tone" proved sufficient to elicit anxiety, with the absence of a smile and the context of a session escalating it further. Rita's therapist provided some exposure to this cue by beginning their sessions with a variety of questions about treatment progress while using a serious tone and not smiling. This exposure did help Rita habituate to the cue in the context of individual therapy, but it had a limited capacity for generalization. Because of the difficulty with arranging in vivo exposure with various "authorities" on the unit, Rita and her therapist decided to use imagery for additional exposure. Rita first imagined a variety of authorities on the unit speaking with serious tones and asking her questions about her progress. She then imagined similar scenarios occurring during scheduled sessions and then added the absence of a smile.

Effective exposure also requires that the client fully participate in experiencing the cue and the emotion. The emotion need not decrease to zero for exposure to change conditioned responses, but clients need to continue the experience until the emotion has decreased notably. Though DBT favors graduated exposure over flooding, the exposure must involve sufficient intensity and duration for learning to occur. For example, Zelda had to remain in the same room as her husband rather than leaving the room to escape from the cue of her husband talking with other women. When Susan's therapist treated the avoidance of the diary card with exposure, she discovered that Susan rushed through completing the diary card in order to minimize exposure to the cue. To ensure full exposure and maximum learning, Susan's therapist would stop Susan whenever she noticed Susan rushing through the card and request that Susan complete the card more slowly and thoughtfully. To treat Dolores's TIBs resulting from the therapist's announcements of trips, the therapist not only presented the cue as often as reasonable, she also extended the duration of the cue by describing in detail the backup arrangements for the client. Without clear instructions and close assessment by therapists, however, clients often fail to achieve the optimum level of exposure. As in traditional exposure therapies, the suboptimum level sometimes results from a lack of clarity about the cue. More often it results from clients avoiding or distracting from the cue, in which case the therapist would add the distraction to the list of behaviors to block.

Many clients expose themselves to more than the intended cue. During the application of exposure to treat Susan's noncompliance of the diary card, her therapist discovered that not only did the cue of "impulsive sex" on the diary card prompt Susan's memory of impulsive sex during that week, those memories then prompted memories of more distal impulsive sex and memories of other "shameful" behaviors. Each memory became a new cue that elicited ever more intense shame. Such a sequence of memories creates the equivalent of someone with a spider phobia handling a spider that starts giving birth to an infinite number of spiders. Similarly, Dolores initially thought about everyone who had ever left her whenever her therapist informed her of a scheduled trip, thus escalating the sadness that she felt about the therapist's absence. In both of these cases, the clients' therapists coached the clients on how to remain mindfully focused on the present cue alone, namely, the current week's diary card for Susan and the therapist's trip for Dolores.

When either the client or the therapist disrupts the exposure to the cue, the therapist treats the reason for the disruption and then re-presents the cue. In Susan's case, any time she appeared to freeze during the exposure, her therapist reminded her to remain mindful of the current week's behavior. If this reminder failed to focus Susan's attention on the current cue, her therapist then paused the exposure to coach Susan on how to implement mindfulness. After this, they would then return to completing the "impulsive sex" column on the diary card. To assess distractions or other deviations from the present cue, many therapists find it useful to have clients describe their experiences aloud during the exposure trial. This practice allows therapists to detect deviations quickly, then to block or shape the deviation accordingly, and finally to return to the presentation of the cue. Describing the experience aloud, however, can also have the effect of slightly distracting clients from the cue, so this practice may work best as a method of assessment rather than as standard practice.

In addition to ensuring the client's exposure to the cue, the therapist and client must also block the client's associated behaviors. Effective response prevention extends beyond blocking obvious, overt behaviors and includes both covert cognitive behaviors and more subtle overt behaviors, such as facial expression, body posture, and verbal expressions. In Jack's case, he and his therapist obviously needed to block his main TIBs of yelling at the therapist and threatening to complain to the therapist's manager. Blocking these behaviors alone, however, would not provide full response prevention. Jack also clenched his jaw and fists and tensed his body. He judged his therapist and ruminated on how he would "not let her get away with this." In Dolores's case, her obvious overt behaviors consisted of phoning the therapist too frequently between sessions, begging the therapist not to leave, and sobbing extensively. Also of relevance, however, Dolores curled her body in the chair while sobbing and repeatedly thought, "Everyone leaves me; nobody cares about me."

Though therapists often cannot block clients' emotional behaviors directly during exposure, they can try not to reinforce those behaviors that occur within their therapeutic context and coach clients on how to notice and prevent the behaviors themselves, particularly by acting opposite to the emotional urges. Jack's therapist, for example, did not reinforce Jack's yelling or threatening by changing to Jack's agenda. If Jack began to engage in either of these behaviors, his therapist would remind him of their exposure plan and its connection to his long-term goals, and then return the focus to the original session task. His therapist also highlighted any time that Jack clenched his fists or jaw and taught him to act opposite while presented with the cue of the therapist's refusal to distract from the session's primary task. The therapist considered progressive relaxation to decrease the tensing, but decided that this procedure would distract from the cue for too long. With respect to the cognitive behaviors, his therapist encouraged Jack to notice his judgmental and other angry thoughts and to describe the facts instead. Dolores's therapist did not change her travel plans in response to Dolores's pleas, nor did she accept phone calls beyond her normal limits. Furthermore, the therapist did not offer reassurance about her return date or their relationship as a consequence of the phone calls, pleas, or tears. Instead, when Dolores started sobbing, the therapist would first stop the sobbing by instructing Dolores to regulate her breathing, and then return to the details of the trip. Similarly, when Dolores begged the therapist to cancel a trip, the therapist would block the behavior by raising her hand and firmly saying "Stop." She would then return to presenting the cue. With respect to telephone contact, they decided that the therapist would not answer more than a specified number of calls during the week as a whole and that any call would end if Dolores started to beg her therapist to stay. Furthermore, the exposure trials required Dolores to act opposite to her urges and to approach rather than avoid the stimuli by asking socially appropriate questions about the proposed trip and by anticipating and generating solutions for any problems that might arise during the therapist's absence. As these cases illustrate, if the prevention of the response has interfered with the presentation of the cue, the therapist and client address the problem and then return to the cue.

Common Problems

Failing to Include Exposure

Perhaps the most common problem is the failure to include exposure as part of the solution analysis when it would likely prove an effective solution. Failing to generate exposure as a potential solution sometimes occurs because of conceptual errors during the BCA or solution analysis. Regular reviews of solution analyses by the consultation team can help to detect and correct conceptual errors that omit exposure. For example, Rita's therapist had previously conducted a similar BCA with Rita, during which she had conceptualized the anger as the key problematic variable. The therapist, therefore, focused the solution analysis on skills to decrease Rita's anger. Rita initially did not collaborate at all, insisting that she "was right" and that the skills "wouldn't change anything." As Rita frequently engaged in such noncollaborative behavior, the therapist did not analyze it and instead pursued the rehearsal of solutions for the anger. Rita agreed to try the solutions, but the commitment seemed weak. During a discussion of the solution analysis at the consultation meeting, another therapist wondered whether the anger in the chain served a particular function that reinforced Rita for maintaining rather than changing the anger. Rita's therapist had not focused on the preceding anxiety because the TIB had occurred after the anger, but she now wondered whether the anger functioned to help Rita avoid the conversation with the psychiatrist and the anxiety. Thus, the next time a similar chain occurred, the therapist pursued this hypothesis and suggested exposing to the cues that elicited anxiety while blocking all escape behaviors. In this instance, the escape behaviors included all of the anger responses, such as making negative assumptions about others, cursing, and threatening to complain. Though Rita did not relish the idea of exposing herself to the relevant cues, she had more motivation to implement this solution because it connected better to her long-term goals. She still tried to avoid the cue through angry responses during the initial in-session trials, but she collaborated with her therapist on trying to block the behaviors and expose herself to the cue. Eventually, she even practiced approaching the cue by asking staff in "authority" what they thought about her treatment progress.

Though conceptual errors sometimes explain the omission of exposure, therapists also often fail to suggest exposure because their own emotions inhibit them. Although these therapists sometimes hesitate to use exposure because they feel guilty about eliciting clients' aversive emotions, they more often fear that the implementation will go awry. In particular, they fear that the client's emotions will escalate beyond a tolerable level and that the client will return to the target behavior. As with any other solution, exposure can go awry for either conceptual or strategic reasons, but when correctly implemented, the brain naturally habituates to the cue and the emotion decreases. Occasionally, therapists inadvertently attempt to implement exposure for an emotion warranted both by type and intensity. In such cases, the emotion will probably not weaken, and the conditioned relationship between the cue and emotion will likely strengthen. Though any therapist can make this error during solution evaluation, therapists who have recently learned to apply exposure sometimes have a particular vulnerability to suggesting exposure for any emotional link. If therapists avoid exposure because they fear suggesting it in the wrong situation, they can solve this problem by reviewing a solution analysis with the consultation team before implementing exposure with the client. More often, therapists engage in one of the common problems described later in this section. In such instances, clients may experience exposure as an ineffective solution, but they most likely will not become overwhelmed by the emotion. To reduce the likelihood of a therapist making such errors, the consultation team can clarify the therapist's conceptualization, review session recordings and role-play relevant strategies. To reduce the fear, however, therapists generally need to use exposure themselves by exposing themselves to a client's escalating emotions, tolerating their own increased fear, and blocking their own fear-based behaviors while implementing the solution with a client.

Erroneously Differentiating Exposure Elements

Exposure sometimes becomes confusing for the therapist and the client because the therapist has insufficiently or inaccurately differentiated the components of exposure (i.e., cue, emotion, and behaviors). Chains that involve primary and secondary emotions particularly increase the difficulty of differentiating the components of exposure. In these chains, the situation often warrants the first emotion but not the second emotion. If the elements of the first emotion have become the cue that elicits the second emotion, then treatment would involve exposing the client to the cue of the first emotion while blocking the behaviors associated with the second emotion. For example, in the case of Jamie, the adolescent who swore at her teachers, her therapist initially thought that the teachers' challenges directly elicited the anger, but then discovered that warranted, moderate shame actually controlled the unwarranted, intense anger. As anger had become a maladaptive response to experiencing shame, Jamie and her therapist developed an exposure hierarchy that involved presenting the elements of shame as the cue, experiencing the emotion of anger rise and fall, and preventing anger-related responses. The shame elements included the sensation of warmth from blushing, a sense of "all eyes upon her," and an urge to withdraw. The obvious, overt responses to prevent included denying the disruptive behavior, raising her voice tone, judging, and swearing at the teacher. Subtle or covert behaviors to block included tensing her body and covertly judging the teacher.

Cueing Errors

Problematic presentations of a cue often can explain why a series of exposure trials have failed to alter the relationship between the stimulus and the emotion. If the therapist or client presents a cue from too high in the exposure hierarchy, the client may experience too much emotional intensity and escape from the cue. In one case, the therapist and client developed a graduated exposure hierarchy for the client's fear, but the client became so excited about overcoming her fear that she started at the top of the hierarchy, quickly felt overwhelmed by her fear, and abandoned her exposure program for that week. After analyzing the TIB in the next session, the client returned to implementing her exposure program, as prescribed this time. Alternatively, exposure may have an insufficient impact if the client does not have a sufficient experience of the cue or conditioned emotion. This can occur for several reasons. If the therapist and client have not adequately identified the cue's components and context, the exposure may miss a critical aspect of the cue. If the intensity of the cue's presentation remains too low, it may not elicit enough emotional intensity. If the duration of the cue occurs too briefly, the client may not experience a sufficient rise or fall in the emotion. This tends to happen if the client becomes distracted from or otherwise unmindful of the cue and then does not return to it. Jane's case illustrates several of the potential cueing problems. When she and her therapist initially targeted bingeing, Jane tried to avoid the analyses because of shame unwarranted by its intensity. Although Jane experienced notably more unwarranted shame while analyzing the bingeing than the suicidal behaviors or vomiting, her therapist initially tried to use very informal exposure by simply continuing with the BCA, as this solution had succeeded with the other targets. Unfortunately, the shame response did not decrease. After watching a portion of a recorded therapy session, the consultation team wondered whether the therapist may have missed an aspect of the cue. In particular, one member of the team noticed that Jane's shame seemed to increase when she briefly described the binge itself and then decreased when they proceeded to identify links in the chain. When the therapist discussed this with Jane, they discovered that the most critical cue for the unwarranted intensity of shame was the memory in general and visualization in particular of exactly what and how much she ate and how she ate it. To expose Jane to this critical set of cues, her therapist requested that Jane imagine herself in her kitchen and then describe the relevant details of target binges before they proceeded to the chain analysis itself. This strategy seemed to have some success but not as much as expected. When the therapist listened to the beginning of the recorded session, she realized that Jane sped through the detailed description. To correct this, the therapist stopped Jane any time that she noticed Jane speeding through a description and then asked Jane to start the description from the beginning. Jane's shame quickly reduced after applying this strategy. Though discussions with clients or consultation teams can help therapists to detect cueing problems, the therapist or team may not have enough information to analyze the problem. In-session or in vivo trials with the therapist present may provide the best opportunity for therapists to assess the client's cueing problems. Role plays during consultation team can help to detect the therapist's cueing errors, but listening to recorded sessions often provides a better opportunity to detect the therapist's and client's errors alike.

Failing to Block Associated Behaviors

Failing to block behaviors associated with the emotion can also explain the continuation of conditioned emotional and behavioral responses. Often, comprehensive response prevention does not occur because the therapist and client have not thoroughly assessed and identified the behaviors to block. Cognitions, facial expressions, subtle body posture, and some verbal communications seem more vulnerable to neglect than targets or other overt behaviors. In Carmella's case, she and her therapist initially focused on stopping her from avoiding skills training sessions and work days. With the aid of telephone coaching from her therapist, Carmella immediately stopped missing groups and decreased missing work, but her shame in these contexts did not decrease. When she raised this problem with the consultation team, one of the skills trainers highlighted that Carmella sometimes sat in group with her head down, even when reporting on her homework or practicing a new skill, and spoke in a quieter voice than usual. When the therapist assessed these behaviors during individual therapy, Carmella acknowledged that she intentionally looked down when experiencing shame because of worsened acne, both at group and work, but she had not noticed speaking more softly. This more thorough assessment also revealed that in these contexts, she often stopped attending to others and instead imagined herself at home. After Carmella began blocking these behaviors as well, her shame decreased in these contexts.

To decrease the likelihood of missing a relevant response, therapists and clients can review the elements of the emotion and assess whether the client engages in any of those elements. As with cueing problems, in-session or in vivo trials with the therapist present may provide the best opportunity for therapists to assess the behaviors to block. Because of the subtle aspects of many overt behaviors, reviewing session recordings can prove essential as well as useful.

CHAPTER 7

COGNITIVE MODIFICATION

KEY PRINCIPLES AND STRATEGIES

Traditionally, behavioral and cognitive models of psychotherapy have maintained different theoretical positions regarding the degree to which cognitions control or mediate emotions and overt behaviors. Beck has described his cognitive therapy (Beck, Rush, Shaw, & Emery, 1979) as "based on a theory of personality which maintains that how one thinks largely determines how one feels and behaves" (Beck & Weishaar, 1989, p. 285). Ellis assigned the following role to cognition in the treatment that he developed (e.g., Ellis & Dryden, 2007): "When a highly charged emotional consequence follows a significant activating event (A), A may seem to but actually does not cause C. Instead, emotional consequences are largely created by B—the individual's belief system" (Ellis, 1989, p. 197). In the decades since Beck and Ellis introduced their treatments, many studies have supported their theoretical position of cognitions as causal. In contrast, Skinner (1976, p. 115) said of cognitive processes or covert behavior, "Covert behavior is also easily observed and by no means unimportant. . . . It would also be a mistake not to recognize its limitations. . . . It does not explain overt behavior: it is simply more behavior to be explained." Behaviorists question the extent to which one can infer causality from chronology. They would argue that just because a thought occurs immediately before an action, it does not follow that the thought caused the action. Like the overt behavior, the covert behavior may occur as another consequence of the preceding stimulus and without any causal or mediating impact of its own. Susan, for example, reported that immediately after she thought "I don't even deserve to live," she noticed an increased impulse to self-harm. The judgment could have caused the increased impulse, but equally the preceding guilt could have caused both the judgment and the impulse, with the impulse simply entering conscious awareness more slowly than the thought.

DBT maintains a dialectical position in the debate regarding the causal or mediating impact of cognitions. While conducting BCAs, therapists highlight potentially problematic cognitions, in terms of both thought content (e.g., "I'm evil," "He's doing that because he doesn't like me," "Why did I do that? If only I hadn't, everything would be fine!") and types of thinking (e.g., judging, interpreting, ruminating, remembering). Therapists then analyze whether those cognitions contribute causally to target behaviors or simply occur as epiphenomena. Sometimes, the solution analysis helps to clarify causality. For example, one client easily and convincingly challenged her thought "He'll never come back," but changing this thought had no impact on her anxiety about her husband "storming" out of the house. On the antecedent side of the BCA, cognitions may initiate or increase behavioral impulses directly, or they may elicit or exacerbate an emotion that then motivates a behavior. For example, in the BCA of Jane's vomiting, the thought "Mom's right. I'm selfish, hopeless, and too focused on myself" appears to elicit guilt directly, as nothing in Jane's previous BCAs suggested a classically conditioned response between guilt and either "fat," fear or shame. Cognitions may also motivate target behaviors when they occur on the consequence side. For example, decreased guilt reinforced both Jane's and Susan's target behaviors, but their decreased guilt appeared to depend partly on the belief that their respective target behavior had sufficiently "punished" them. Though the treatment of cognitions in DBT includes the application of traditional cognitive therapy strategies, the treatment's theoretical foundations result in different conceptual and strategic emphases. The first section of this chapter describes the distinctive features of treating cognitions in DBT and reviews the application of standard cognitive procedures. The remainder of the chapter discusses common problems in applying cognitive procedures in DBT.

Distinctive DBT Features

The biosocial, behavioral, and dialectical principles of DBT all contribute to the distinction between DBT and traditional cognitive therapy approaches to treating cognitive processes. Because the biosocial theory emphasizes the role that emotion plays in the motivation to engage in target behaviors, DBT therapists particularly attend to emotion links in the BCA and solution analysis. Indeed, a lack of attention to emotions will reduce therapists' adherence scores, whereas a lack of attention to cognitive links need not impact adherence. In Rita's solution analysis, the therapist generated solutions for an approximately equal number of emotions and cognitions, but she and Rita spent notably more time implementing the solution for the emotions. During their respective solution analyses, Susan and Jane each spent more time generating and rehearsing solutions for their emotions than for their cognitions.

Behavioral theories influence both how DBT conceptualizes cognition as a controlling variable and how it explains the development and, more importantly, the maintenance of maladaptive thinking. Similar to Linehan's (1993a) biosocial theory, behavioral approaches do not prioritize cognition as a mediating variable, instead they consider the stimulus, emotional response, and contingencies as quite significant. Relative to approaches that include constructs such as "schemas" (e.g., Beck et al., 1979), behavioral theory emphasizes process over structure. Thus, therapists do not search for a "core" belief, but instead analyze each thought in terms of how much it influenced emotions and actions in that moment, as well as how frequently it occurs. The emphasis on maladaptive thinking as learned behavior differentiates DBT from Ellis's treatment (e.g., Ellis, 1989; Ellis & Dryden, 2007), which proposes an inherent tendency toward "irrational beliefs." Furthermore, DBT analyzes the function of cognitive behaviors to understand their maintenance, especially when clients have refused to try cognitive solutions or traditional cognitive therapy techniques have not changed the cognition. Functional consequences often maintain maladaptive covert behaviors, as well as overt behaviors. For example, many suicidal clients experience a reinforcing decrease in aversive emotions simply by fantasizing about suicide. Swann's research on self-verification (Swann et al., 1992) describes how validating thoughts also function to reduce arousal. Some clients engage in patterns of thinking often referred to as "permission-giving" thoughts. These thoughts commonly occur when clients have urges to engage in target or other problematic behaviors, but emotions or other cognitions inhibit any action. "Permission-giving" thoughts function to reduce the inhibition, most commonly guilt or shame. Ultimately, if the therapy does not address the function of a cognitive behavior under operant control, the cognition will likely persist, regardless of any attempts to modify it.

Conceptualizing cognitions as operant behaviors introduces contingency management as another type of solution for problematic cognitive links controlled partly by their consequences. From a contingency management perspective, therapists can decrease a cognitive behavior by punishing it, by removing its reinforcing consequence, or by shaping a skillful behavior that better achieves the cognitive behavior's function. Though any challenge to a cognitive behavior, whether asking for supporting evidence or labeling it as irrational, may punish the behavior, such punishment would more likely suppress the expression of the thought rather than the thought itself. DBT therapists instead emphasize removing reinforcing consequences and shaping skillful behaviors to address the function.

Jane repeatedly fantasized about suicide, with a particular focus on how suicide would allow her to "escape" from her problems and her mother would "be better off" if she died. When her therapist initially attempted to use traditional cognitive techniques to decrease this fantasizing, Jane dismissed the solutions by saying "That won't work." Because Jane had successfully used these techniques previously and she dismissed them so quickly this time, the therapist suspected that the cognitions served a particular function. When the therapist asked what would happen if Jane did stop fantasizing, Jane responded that she would "have no escape." The therapist then focused on the function of fantasizing about suicide and learned that the behavior functioned to decrease Jane's anxiety about current problems, physical tension related to the anxiety, and guilt about the amount of care her mother provided her. Thus, the immediate emotional and physiological relief that Jane experienced when fantasizing about suicide shaped suicidal thinking via negative reinforcement. The therapist's initial plan was to have Jane challenge her thought that her mother would "be better off" by examining the evidence. This presumably would remove the reinforcement for the thought and might even punish it by showing that Jane would have even more to feel guilty about if she committed suicide. Jane refused to try this cognitive restructuring, however, because she had more motivation to maintain the fantasizing than to change it. Thus, her therapist decided first to focus on blocking reinforcement of suicidal thinking in session while shaping Jane's use of skills that could achieve the emotion regulation function of the fantasizing. Therefore, whenever Jane reported thinking that suicide would lead to "escape" from her problems or to her mother "being better off," the therapist attempted to block a consequent decrease in anxiety, tension, or guilt. The therapist would sit forward in her chair and with a serious facial expression would say extremely firmly, "STOP. No Jane, killing yourself IS NOT a solution. It's a MAJOR problem. Your mother will be devastated. We have to find a real solution." Next, the therapist reviewed the evidence of the impact of suicide on relatives and highlighted that many of the world's major faiths dispute the idea that suicide solves problems. The therapist and Jane then focused on generating and implementing a range of skillful behaviors to decrease her tension and regulate her emotions. Although Jane disliked the blocking and challenging of her beliefs, after experiencing these strategies several times in session, she reported that whenever suicidal thoughts arose she first envisaged the therapist saying "STOP! No, this is a problem," and then thought about using other solutions. After Jane had experienced the more skillful solutions as helpful in decreasing her physical tension and regulating her emotions, she became more willing to apply traditional cognitive restructuring herself.

Dialectical principles guide therapists to balance the traditional cognitive-behavioral emphasis on changing cognitions with an emphasis on acceptance. To achieve this balance, therapists validate clients' cognitions in the current context and include acceptance-oriented strategies (e.g., mindfulness, wise mind, radical acceptance, self-validation) in the solution analysis. Therapists and clients may validate cognitive processes as normal in the current context (as opposed to past learning). For example, most people spend time judging, assuming, worrying, and ruminating. Alternatively, therapists and clients can validate cognitions by validating their function. In Jane's case, fantasizing about suicide had validity in that it effectively functioned to decrease aversive emotions. When warranted by the facts, therapists also validate the content of clients' thoughts, even if the content elicits problematic emotional or behavioral responses. When Susan reported thinking "I'm a cheat," her therapist agreed with her because factually Susan had cheated repeatedly. When the thought occurred in another chain, the therapist again validated the content and then proceeded to analyze solutions for the link, as it seemed to contribute to Susan's suicidality. The therapist's direct and immediate validation on both occasions increased Susan's willingness to collaborate and to try radical acceptance as a solution. Had her therapist challenged the thought instead, Susan likely would have become less collaborative, focused instead on proving her point. Ultimately of course, solving Susan's problems required her to change her cheating rather than her thinking.

After several episodes of aggressive behavior on the ward, Rita stated, "The staff don't like me and want me to leave." As the therapist had heard such sentiments about Rita expressed by staff, she validated the general accuracy of Rita's belief. She also highlighted that Rita could change the way that staff thought about her by stopping her aggressive behavior, as the staff members' opinions resulted directly from that behavior. Similar to Susan, Rita's aggressive behavior had to change before her belief that others disliked her changed.

Regardless of the validity of cognitions, therapists can use acceptance-based skills to treat cognitions that mediate or control emotions or target behaviors. Though a variety of skills, such as wise mind and radical acceptance, involve acceptance as a component, therapists tend to suggest mindfulness most frequently for maladaptive cognitions. Though skills training groups teach clients the basics of mindfulness, individual therapists further strengthen these skills by highlighting unmindful thinking whenever it occurs during therapy sessions or appears in chain analyses. They then ask clients to practice more mindful thinking. Mindfulness seems particularly effective in comparison to traditional cognitive restructuring strategies when treating unconditional judgmental thinking, which does not involve facts to prove or disprove.

Judgmental thinking occurred several times in Susan's chain. Early in the chain, she thought "I shouldn't have sex with someone else," then consequently experienced intense guilt. The "should" in such a thought could be conditional, meaning that if Susan desires maintaining her relationship with her boyfriend who values fidelity, then indeed she should not sleep with a stranger as doing so could risk her relationship. In this case, however, further assessment clarified that the thought expressed an unconditional, moral evaluation. Later in the chain, Susan again judged herself, this time as not deserving her boyfriend and not deserving to live, which seemed to further increase her self-harm urges. If her therapist had tried to challenge these cognitions with traditional cognitive restructuring techniques, Susan probably would have supplied plenty of evidence for the rationality of her beliefs, particularly with respect to the judgments about sleeping with strangers and deserving her boyfriend. Instead, her therapist suggested mindfully letting go of the judgmental thoughts. In the first solution analysis, the therapist focused on implementing mindfulness for "I don't even deserve to live," as this seemed the most problematic judgment with respect to suicidal behavior. To let go of the judgment, Susan practiced describing "I don't deserve" as a judgment and then describing the relevant facts, namely, that she had acted against her values and had broken a commitment, that she felt intense guilt and shame, and that she had strong urges to do anything to stop the emotions. She then practiced refocusing her attention on the relevant tasks, particularly on using skills to manage her emotions and preventing herself from overdosing. Subsequent solution analyses for similar chains also included mindfulness for the other judgmental links.

Mindfulness also seems comparatively effective relative to cognitive restructuring when the content of the thought has possible or definite validity, but the context does not warrant the type of thinking. For example, Rita's thoughts about the staff's opinions of her closely resembled the facts, but just ruminating about staff opinions had no adaptive benefit, especially in the middle of a suicidal crisis. Similarly, during interpersonal conflicts Rita tended to ruminate about past episodes of conflict for which she blamed others. Though the attribution of blame to others had validity, ruminating on it interfered with resolving the current conflict. To decrease such ruminating in both situations, her therapist encouraged her to use mindfulness but Rita initially refused. Analyses of these refusals revealed that thinking about the staff not liking her functioned to "give permission" for self-harm, whereas reminding herself of others' blame functioned to decrease her anxiety. After her therapist treated the motivational obstacles to letting go of unmindful thinking, Rita willingly practiced mindfulness.

Standard CBT Procedures

Standard cognitive change procedures generally begin with the identification of a cognition or set of cognitions to change. As in standard CBT, DBT therapists shape clients' abilities to recognize and describe types of cognitive content and processes. Therapists and clients can label cognitions with a range of standard labels (e.g., assuming, biased reasoning, catastrophizing, dichotomous thinking, emotional reasoning, filtering, and mood dependent). They can also create their own labels. The choice of label depends on what will best help clients to identify problematic cognitions or generate matching solutions. For example, clients who think "I can't" as a way to give themselves permission not to try a skill often label these thoughts as "permission giving" because they have learned that labeling the function of the thought often mitigates the thought's impact, as well as directing them toward using cognitive restructuring. In contrast, clients who think "I can't" because they have confused an interpretation with a description can benefit from labeling the thought as an interpretation. This label will suggest the cognitive restructuring strategies of examining the evidence and generating alterative interpretations. Though DBT therapists only prescribe formal thought records as needed, they have ample opportunity to highlight problematic cognitions that occur in chains leading to target behaviors or that occur during the session. After highlighting problematic cognition, therapists usually either teach newer clients how to notice and label the cognition or ask more advanced clients to label it themselves. In some instances, labeling leads directly to the client stopping the problematic thinking. For example, one client quickly corrected overgeneralized thinking as soon as either she or the therapist had identified it. In other instances, however, the therapist may need to apply additional cognitive restructuring procedures. With the same client for example, just labeling potentially inaccurate interpretations did not alter them, so the therapist taught the client both to examine the evidence and generate alternative interpretations. Therapists and clients may either immediately interweave such cognitive restructuring procedures or continue the BCA and possibly return to the cognition during a comprehensive solution analysis.

DBT therapists use a variety of CBT procedures to change cognitions. The most commonly used include challenging maladaptive cognitions, Socratic debating, examining the evidence or experimenting to gather evidence, generating alternative thoughts, shaping dialectical thinking, clarifying contingencies, and providing didactic information. These procedures can vary in their emphasis on decreasing maladaptive cognitions versus increasing adaptive cognitions, on changing the content of thoughts versus the type of thinking, and the degree to which they require knowledge of the facts.

Challenging, debating, examining the evidence, and experimenting all aim to disrupt clients' problematic cognitions. Challenging refers to directly communicating to clients that they have engaged in problematic thinking, whereas Socratic debate indirectly reveals the problems through questioning that eventually reveals the contradictions or lack of logic in clients' thinking. Examining the evidence and conducting experiments to gather evidence more actively involve clients in the change process. Using either of these interventions effectively requires accurate assessment by therapists that the content of the cognitions most likely will prove inaccurate or otherwise faulty. For example, Jane's therapist never suggested examining the evidence when Jane thought that her brother had left the family home because of Jane's behavior, as the therapist knew that Jane could produce extensive evidence for this belief, including letters in which the brother had expressed this. Jane and her therapist decided to use radical acceptance and "focusing on the present" as solutions instead. Earlier in the chain when Jane thought "I'm always going to be fat" and "I have no control," examining the evidence eventually proved helpful. Although Jane produced a notable amount of evidence for "no control," she also identified several aspects of her current situation over which she had some control, such as choosing which skills to use, selecting television programs to watch, and deciding whether or not to try on clothing or study herself in mirrors. Reviewing the evidence helped Jane to decrease the intensity of her belief that she had no control. Through examining the evidence, Jane also changed the cognition "Now I'm in control" that occurred after vomiting, especially when she reviewed the evidence that most people would evaluate her vomiting as indicating an absence of control.

As with other behaviors, clients generally have better success in decreasing a dysfunctional cognitive behavior if they simultaneously engage in an incompatible cognitive behavior. For example, to decrease judgmental thinking, therapists do not simply tell clients to "Let go of judgments." Instead, they teach clients how to develop mindful thinking that involves describing judgments as judgments and attending to the facts of their current context. Similarly, DBT therapists, like therapists using many other CBT models, often pair decreasing dichotomous or extreme thinking with increasing some degree of dialectical thinking. To decrease Jane's extreme thinking (e.g., "I have no control"), her therapist shaped her dialectical thinking. Examining the evidence started this process by identifying and validating two sides to the debate, but it did not create any syntheses. Searching for syntheses created the new thought "I can't control all factors that influence my behavior. If I use skills regularly, however, I'll have fewer things that I need to control." Developing dialectical thinking processes also revealed the paradox "Sometimes, trying to control everything leads to losing control." Jane initially found it more difficult to think dialectically than to examine the evidence for her thoughts, but she eventually found that dialectical thinking generalized to a wider variety of situations because it shifted her attention away from her thinking and toward engaging skillfully in the task at hand. After Rita spontaneously generated a more dialectical statement for "People never understand me," her therapist further shaped dialectical thinking by first asking Rita to describe both sides of the debate and then helping her to search for a synthesis. Through this process, Rita created several new thoughts, namely, "How well people understand me varies a lot"; "Their understanding depends on my behavior as much as it does them"; and "When people understand me better, they may do things that I don't like, as well as things that I do like." These thoughts both improved Rita's motivation to engage more effectively with the psychiatrist and diminished her desire for understanding.

When the content rather than the type of thinking seems more problematic, clients can change their cognitions by generating adaptive or alternative thoughts that contradict the maladaptive thoughts. Clients can use this solution when they have identified their interpretations, beliefs about causal relationships, predictions or similar cognitions as faulty, and alternative interpretations, beliefs, or predictions have more known accuracy. If clients do not have sufficient evidence to determine the accuracy of their thoughts or they either cannot or will not attempt to gather evidence, they can still use this solution to weaken the intensity of or their attachment to the maladaptive thought. For example, because interpretations of other people's behaviors often have emotional and behavioral consequences, therapists often focus on reducing inaccurate interpretations. Unfortunately, clients sometimes lack both the information required to assess an interpretation's accuracy and the opportunity to investigate it further. In such circumstances, clients can still generate alternative interpretations and compare the probable accuracy of all interpretations. Even if this exercise does not identify a more probable alternative, it may still decrease the attachment to the original interpretation. Although clients may have acquired the basics of this technique during the emotion regulation skills training module, individual therapy further strengthens the technique by generating and rehearsing it in session as a solution for specific interpretations leading to specific target behaviors.

In a later chain analysis in Rita's case, when the psychiatrist asked, "How do you feel things are going here?" Rita again thought "He thinks I'm getting worse, that I don't deserve to be here." This time, she immediately reminded herself that she had no evidence to support this interpretation, but as she could not think of any other explanation, this interpretation returned. She thought about asking her psychiatrist about her interpretation, but experienced too much inhibition to ask and doubted that she would believe him anyway. Therefore, as part of the solution analysis, her therapist helped Rita to generate as many interpretations as she could about the reason for her psychiatrist's inquiry. Rita's alternative interpretations included "He thinks I'm a hopeless case," "He hasn't read up about my case," "He's wondering if they should do different things to help," "He's thinking about increasing my observation levels," and "He's interested in my opinion." She noticed that while she generated more interpretations, she forgot her original interpretation. Rita and her therapist then considered the relative merits of the interpretations, both in terms of accuracy and effectiveness. She could not differentiate the cognitions based on accuracy, but could easily differentiate their effectiveness. At this point, the therapist contributed what she knew about the psychiatrist both to enhance accuracy and to reinforce Rita's efforts. Based on her knowledge, the therapist thought it most likely that the psychiatrist wondered what else the staff team could do to help or had a genuine interest in Rita's opinion or both. In addition to directly teaching clients how to generate alternative interpretations, therapists can model this technique by cultivating genuine nonattachment to their own interpretations. Thus, Rita's therapist mindfully described her own ideas as interpretations rather than facts.

A lack of attention to or knowledge about causal relationships also causes problems. Clients frequently remain unaware of the impact of their behavior on themselves and others, as well as about causal rules in general. For example, many clients with eating disorders do not realize that starving can interfere with losing weight. Through contingency clarification, DBT therapists aim to increase attention to and accuracy of beliefs about causal relationships in order to shift clients' motivation. Therapists highlight and have clients practice identifying the "if–then" rules that operate within clients' lives generally and in therapy particularly. In and of itself, contingency clarification is a form of cognitive modification. This strategy also closely links with contingency management, as the therapist may implement the highlighted contingencies.

During one individual DBT session, Rita threatened to file a formal complaint because her therapist "kept pushing" her to use skills. Rita's therapist then effectively used contingency clarification to decrease Rita's motivation to persist with this TIB. When the therapist asked what Rita thought would happen as a consequence of threatening to complain, Rita stated that she thought her therapist would "listen" to her, stop "talking about skills," and stop "demanding so much." The therapist clarified that although the threat did increase her general level of attentiveness, it also distracted her from attending to Rita's problems and toward attending to how she could protect herself. She also highlighted that while this focus on protecting herself from the threat might lead to decreased demands for skills use, it might also lead to a decrease in her motivation or ability to help Rita. When the therapist asked what Rita expected would happen as a consequence of actually filing a complaint, Rita replied that she expected management to tell the therapist to stop asking about and suggesting skills. The therapist then clarified that before taking such action, the management first would need to investigate the complaint and might prevent the therapist from working with Rita during the course of the investigation. If they did tell the therapist not to use skills as a solution, then the therapist could not continue therapy with Rita, as she could not conduct effective DBT with such restrictions. The therapist also clarified the consequences of management deciding against the complaint, including the risk that Rita may become viewed as a chronic complainer and taken less seriously in the future. Rita stated that she really did not want to lose her therapist or to be dismissed as a chronic complainer and revealed that her motivation to complain formally decreased when she considered these consequences. To strengthen the association between filing a complaint about the emphasis on skills and the possible outcomes that Rita did not want, Rita's therapist had Rita imagine filing a complaint and then experiencing these consequences. After this session, when Rita had urges to complain formally or threaten her therapist with complaints, she also would remember the in-session contingency clarification. Her motivation to threaten then would decline dramatically. Of course, the therapist also generated solutions for other variables that controlled the threatening, including interpersonal skills that Rita could use to alert her therapist whenever the therapist oversimplified the task of learning or implementing skills.

Like standard CBT therapists, DBT therapists frequently provide didactic information to prevent or correct inaccurate beliefs and to develop more accurate ones. Therapists use information from multiple fields of science, including biology, cognitive science, and behavioral learning. For example, Jane's therapist provided information about the perceptual distortions of body image common to clients with eating disorders and the impact of culture on perceptions of beauty and body shape. Jane used this information to challenge both some of her perceptions of her body and her long-held beliefs about the importance of weight, shape, and body image. For Carmella, learning about confirmation biases increased her awareness of this type of cognitive bias and her motivation to shift her attention to assessing rather than confirming her beliefs. Susan's therapist provided information about the technical definitions of reinforcement and punishment to restructure Susan's thought that spending time in the hospital after her overdose "was a punishment." This information helped Susan to clarify the contingencies of the hospital stay, which functioned to reduce her guilt rather than punish her infidelity. She then stopped thinking that she had "punished herself," and consequently no longer experienced relief from her guilt through overdosing.

COMMON PROBLEMS

As with other solutions, problems with cognitive modification commonly result from strategic nonadherence, conceptual errors, or a combination of the two, sometimes exacerbated by therapists' motivational issues or clients' TIBs. Problems can occur during any step in the solution analysis, though therapists seem to have more difficulties with the generation and implementation of cognitive solutions than their evaluation. In contrast to the underuse of exposure highlighted in Chapter 6, the overuse of cognitive modification seems to occur at least as often as its underuse. Listening to session recordings and role playing generally provides teams with the best opportunities to identify these problems if the therapist has not done so already, though reviews of written solution analyses often proves efficient for the more conceptual problems. This next section divides the common problems of cognitive modification into those more closely associated with standard CBT treatments and those more associated with key DBT elements.

CBT Procedures

Failing to Teach the Client to Label Cognitions

Not teaching clients how to label problematic cognitions decreases their ability to identify the cognitions and to generate corresponding solutions. Although the problem can occur if therapists conduct chain analyses unmindfully and thus fail to recognize relevant links, some therapists, especially those without previous training in CBT or mindfulness, lack the ability to identify certain cognitive problems or to discriminate effectively among types of cognitive problems. For example, therapists commonly confuse judgmental judgments as described in the DBT skills manual (Linehan, 1993b) with the colloquial use of the term "judgment" or with statements of preference. In such instances, therapists may confuse or even invalidate clients and generate less effective or even ineffective solutions. One therapist consistently mislabeled the client's statements of "I can't" as judgmental and thus never considered using cognitive restructuring to examine the evidence for the statement. When another therapist complained about her client's noncollaborative response to having judgmental statements highlighted, the team discovered that the therapist had consistently mislabeled the client's statements of dislikes as judgments, thus invalidating the client. In both of these cases, the team recommended more mindfulness training for the therapists. Therapists who have difficulty labeling other types of cognitive processes (e.g., catastrophic thinking, dichotomous thinking) might find lists of these types of thinking helpful.

Other therapists readily recognize clients' problematic cognitions, but they sometimes hesitate to label certain cognitions. In such instances, a brief analysis will reveal what combination of the therapists' own cognitions (e.g., "It's mean to keep highlighting that she's using emotional reasoning"), emotions (e.g., guilt, fear), and the probable consequences of labeling (e.g., client likely to withdraw or express anger) have inhibited the therapist. With this information, the therapist or team can generate and implement corresponding solutions. For example, one therapist stopped labeling a client's dysfunctional cognitions after the client repeatedly became noncollaborative in response to the labeling. In response to the therapist's request for consultation, the team suggested that the therapist return to labeling and then conduct a brief BCA on the client's TIB. The analysis revealed classically conditioned intense, unwarranted shame as a key controlling variable. As this pattern appeared in the analyses to other target behaviors, the therapist and client agreed that it would prove more effective to change the client's response to labeling rather than to stop labeling dysfunctional cognitions.

Substituting Cheerleading or Reassuring for Cognitive Restructuring

Regardless of whether they have labeled a dysfunctional cognition or not, therapists sometimes respond to such cognitions by cheerleading or trying to reassure clients and then assume that they have used cognitive modification strategies. Examples include responding to a client saying, "I can't," with only "Yes, you can," or a client saying, "I'm worried that no one at the wedding will like me," with "I'm sure they will." Although DBT includes cheerleading as a validation strategy, such simplified challenging of clients' beliefs does not equal cognitive modification and risks replicating the oversimplified problem-solving characteristic of invalidating environments (Linehan, 1993a). As with labeling, this problem occurs more often among therapists without basic CBT training. In such instances, role playing with the consultation team can help the therapist acquire and strengthen the skills needed to respond with cognitive restructuring rather than reassurance when required. The problem can also occur if therapists become emotionally dysregulated by clients' beliefs. For example, one therapist reported to her team that when her client said that his children "would be better off" if he "weren't part of their lives," she became very frightened and just repeated "No, that isn't true, they need you," every time the client expressed a similar cognition. Of the solutions that the team generated, the therapist found it most helpful to role-play how to respond with cognitive modification to different team members expressing similar beliefs. This role playing had the effect of both strengthening the therapist's cognitive modification skills and exposing her repeatedly to a cue that had elicited an unwarranted level of fear.

Neglecting the Modification of Cognitive Processes

Some therapists consistently attend to changing the content of clients' cognitions, but neglect to change the style of clients' cognitive processes. This pattern often involves limiting cognitive modification to replacing "negative" content with "positive" content, for example, substituting negative assumptions about the future with positive assumptions, or substituting negative interpretations about a friend's behavior with positive interpretations. In the extreme, a therapist might use simplistic instructions such as "You just need to think positive," though more often, therapists do help clients to develop new content. Although a focus on the content sometimes proves sufficient, successful cognitive modification usually requires attention to cognitive processes or style as well. For example, a comprehensive conceptualization would consider teaching the client how to examine all assumptions objectively or how to refocus attention away from ineffective assuming, rather than just developing positive assumptions. One new therapist had a client whose BCAs frequently included thinking "I don't deserve to get better." The therapist initially described this thought as "dysfunctional" and then proceeded to help the client to identify reasons why she deserved to decrease her suffering and achieve her goals and to replace the thought with "I do deserve to get better." These interventions did not decrease the client's dysfunctional belief, but did decrease her collaboration, as she continuously returned to arguing for her position. Similarly, the client reported that when she tried the solution at home, she "just kept arguing" with herself, a common side effect of cognitive restructuring focused on content. When the therapist asked the team for consultation, they first labeled the thought as judgmental and then role played with the therapist how to teach the client to reorient her thinking from judging herself to describing her behavior and its consequences factually. For this client, a factual description still included a number of "negative" statements, such as "My drug abuse and promiscuity have embarrassed my family," "My siblings want to avoid me," and "I feel ashamed of my drug abuse and promiscuity." Nevertheless, the client collaborated more with this solution and implemented it more often when she had similar "deserve" thoughts, as it better captured "the truth," according to the client.

Missing Components of Solution Implementation

Regardless of whether the client and therapist decide to change cognitive content or processes, cognitive modification will work only if the client implements it. Although cognitive and behavioral theories differ with respect to how much they consider client insight as a sufficient mechanism for change versus client rehearsal as a necessary mechanism for change, cognitive and behavioral treatments traditionally both involve some degree of teaching and rehearsing new cognitive behaviors during and between therapy sessions. A notable number of therapists, however, regularly use strategies that may enhance clients' insight about existing maladaptive cognitions, but then fail to use strategies to enhance clients' practice of new adaptive cognitions. These therapists often fail to teach clients how to use various types of cognitive restructuring techniques or to ask them to practice those techniques in session. Such a situation was described in Chapter 4 where a therapist asked a number of challenging questions that the client answered with "Yes" or "No," but the client did not practice asking the questions. In one case, the therapist repeatedly labeled a client's interpretations and even suggested that the client evaluate the evidence for the interpretations, but they never practiced this in the session. The client reported the following week that cognitive restructuring "didn't work." When the therapist assessed how exactly the client had applied cognitive restructuring, he discovered that the client's implementation contained a substantial number of extreme statements, worry thoughts, and other types of emotional reasoning as evidence.

Therapists may miss components of implementing cognitive solutions for a range of reasons. If a therapist does not know how to teach the solution to or rehearse it with clients, role playing during consultation meetings may prove most helpful. If a therapist confuses partial with full cognitive restructuring, role playing may clarify the difference. As with skills training, therapists may overestimate clients' knowledge of cognitive restructuring techniques or underestimate what they need to do to help clients learn the techniques. In these instances, restructuring therapists' beliefs may prove sufficient. Finally, some therapists minimize implementing components of cognitive modification because they assume that insight will suffice to change cognitions. Fortunately, the consultation team does not need to rely on insight alone to help a therapist change this assumption; they can select solutions from the full range of cognitive modification techniques.

DBT Features

Neglecting Solutions for Noncognitive Variables

In their solution analyses, some therapists have a pattern of relying primarily on solution generation for cognitions and neglecting solutions for other controlling variables, especially affective links. The individual therapist or consultation team can usually detect such a pattern by reviewing the therapist's summary of the solution analysis. This pattern sometimes occurs because the therapist has applied a cognitive theory rather than the biosocial theory to the behavioral conceptualization of the target behavior. More often, therapists focus primarily on cognitive variables and solutions because they learned to do so successfully in other therapy models. The emphasis on cognitions now occurs either automatically or intentionally with little effort or worry compared with newly learned procedures. Some therapists simply need more prompts, in session or from the team, to extend their solution analyses beyond cognitive variables, but other therapists require a more comprehensive set of solutions to address skills deficits and motivational obstacles.

Responding Nondialectically to Cognitions

Therapists sometimes successfully generate solutions for multiple variables in the chain, but respond nondialectically to the cognitive links. One type of nondialectical response involves losing the balance between problem solving and validation. Another type, within problem solving itself, occurs when the solutions for cognitions become too heavily weighted toward either acceptance- or change-based solutions. Individual therapists and consultation teams can often spot these types of nondialectical responses by simply reviewing a solution analysis, though an imbalance between validation and problem solving may only become apparent through listening to sessions or role playing.

One of the most significant mistakes that therapists can make is to invalidate the valid aspects of cognitions. They may treat relatively accurate cognitions as inaccurate by trying to change them with cognitive restructuring, or they may oversimplify the client's experience by dismissing a client's statement as "just a thought." Not only will such solutions likely fail, but the invalidation may lead to an increase in the client's cognitive and emotional dysregulation and a related decrease in the client's learning and collaboration. Therapists sometimes make this error due to their own automatic assumption that any "negative" thought must be faulty and changed. This happened in the case of Jack whose therapist initially invalidated Jack's accurate belief that the staff disliked him. Another therapist initially assumed that her adolescent client, Goa, repeatedly misinterpreted her mother's comments as revealing that her mother did not love her. Whenever the therapist tried cognitive restructuring, the client became angry and stopped collaborating. Only after a family meeting did the therapist realize the accuracy of Goa's interpretation and the extent to which she had invalidated Goa each time she had attempted cognitive restructuring. At other times, therapists may invalidate valid beliefs because of their own emotions about the client's situation or belief. For example, another adolescent client had become disfigured in an accident and now believed that boys would think her unattractive and not want to date her. The therapist validated the normality of such thinking and then immediately proceeded to challenge the belief by highlighting examples of married people with disabilities and describing the importance of "inner beauty," at which point, the client began to cry and to "withdraw" in the session. While most members of the consultation team agreed with the therapist's intervention, a couple suggested that although the therapist had normalized the client's thinking, she had not validated the fact that the client's disfigurement likely would limit her dating options. The therapist acknowledged that when she had thought about the facts of the situation, her sadness and fear of "making it worse" for the client had inhibited her. When she shared this with the client, the client revealed that she had begun crying in the last session because she "felt all alone" because her therapist seemed to imply that her "thoughts were the problem," not the disfigurement itself.

Erring in the opposite direction by validating rather than problem solving faulty cognitions seldom decreases a clients' collaboration, but it does decrease their learning. For example, one client frequently thought "I know that I'm going to binge later," and then stopped trying to decrease her binging urges or block preparations for bingeing. The therapist accepted the client's thought as a statement of fact about the future rather than identifying it as a possible example of the common cognitive error of predicting the future. As a consequence, the therapist missed an opportunity to teach the client how to recognize and correct such errors and to break a potentially important link in the chain.

In the case of Jo-Jo, a client in a forensic substance abuse program, his therapist consistently accepted his statements that he "couldn't" use a particular skill as statements of fact. Consequently, she restricted the solution generation to a few solutions that Jo-Jo said he could use, mainly distress-tolerance skills. After listening to part of the therapist's session, the team asked whether she had assessed the accuracy of Jo-Jo's beliefs about his capabilities. The therapist acknowledged that she had not considered any problem solving for this link, having considered it a statement of fact rather that identifying it as a thought that may or may not reflect the facts. When the therapist and Jo-Jo assessed the accuracy of "couldn't," they discovered that most often Jo-Jo had made an assumption about why he had not used a skill and that "I don't want to use the skill" often would have been more accurate. Cognitive restructuring successfully decreased the frequency of the faulty "I can't" links, but Jo-Jo reported that he then became "stuck" on "I don't want" and a related judgmental rule of "I shouldn't have to do what I don't want." After trying several solutions, the most effective combination included mindfulness for the judgmental rule and self-validation of "don't want" immediately followed by clarifying the contingencies of acting on "wants."

Generating only change-based solutions, such as cognitive restructuring, or only acceptance-based solutions, such as mindfulness or radical acceptance, for maladaptive cognitions also diminishes the dialectical quality of the solution analysis. Chapter 4 provides several examples of underutilizing the change end. In an illustration of the opposite problem, one client interpreted the way that her son said goodbye to her as a sign that he did not care about her. As she ruminated on this, she became convinced that she had "no reason to live." The client and therapist first considered only cognitive restructuring for the initial interpretation and "no reason to live." The cognitive restructuring had some success, but the client also identified substantial evidence to support her original thought. When the team reviewed the solution analysis, they agreed that these solutions matched the links, but suggested that the client might also benefit from mindfulness or radical acceptance. Ultimately, the client found generating alternative interpretations for and radical acceptance of her son's behavior most helpful for the first thought and mindfulness most helpful for ruminating and thinking she had "no reason to live."

Not Applying Behavioral Theory to Cognitions

When treating cognitive links, therapists sometimes fail to apply a behavioral model to their conceptualization of the links. Occasionally, therapists do not apply behavioral theory fully and consequently miss opportunities for change. For example, therapists usually have success using cognitive restructuring and mindfulness for classically conditioned cognitions, but when these techniques fail to modify the cognitions, therapists sometimes forget to consider whether operant conditioning is maintaining the cognitions and whether the treatment needs to address their function. In one case, a client felt intense guilt and shame whenever she failed to fulfill a task as a wife or mother. She would then think "I should be punished" and force herself to vomit. Next, she would think "Now I've punished myself enough" and stop vomiting. Her guilt and shame then decreased. The therapist immediately recognized the first thought as judgmental and coached the client to practice letting go of the judgment. The client demonstrated that she had the skill, but the judgment continued. The therapist then tried examining the evidence and dialectical thinking, but the judgment continued. Meanwhile, the therapist had not attended to the second cognition, which seemed to stop the purging. She did know, however, that the purging primarily functioned to decrease the client's shame and guilt. When the therapist reviewed the solution analysis with the team, they suggested that the "should" might have a function as well, namely, to give the client "permission" to purge, a behavior already motivated by its emotion regulation function. They also suggested that although the second thought may have helped to stop this episode of vomiting, it could actually motivate future episodes if it controlled the decrease in guilt. Based on this new behavioral conceptualization, the therapist introduced contingency clarification and didactic teaching into the solution analysis. More specifically, she clarified the contingent relationship between the thoughts, vomiting, and emotions and taught the client to use the scientific definition of punishment. The client's thinking shifted the most when practicing the following: "There's no evidence that vomiting has ever punished any behaviors and it certainly won't repair the damage that I've done to my family, so there's no reason for me to feel less guilt and shame. If I vomit, it may cause greater distress to my family and warrant more guilt."

Though many therapists occasionally forget to apply an aspect of behavioral theory to treating cognitions, a few therapists tend to switch to a different theoretical model entirely when responding to cognitive variables. For example, they may attend to the function of clients' cognitions, but make assumptions about those functions based on a different theory. This error often leads therapists to severely restrict the range of functions that they consider. Therapists also use a nonbehavioral model when they emphasize insight, particularly into the origins of clients' cognitions, as a primary mechanism of change. This error usually results in an insufficient analysis of the current variables that maintain the cognitions, few solutions for these variables, and little implementation of these solutions. For example, one therapist consistently used Socratic questioning to change the client's cognitions as he believed that insight had to originate within the client for change to occur, but waiting for the client to have insight left little time for other solutions, and the insight itself failed to generalize beyond the session. Finally, conceptualizing some types of cognitions as being "deeper" than others, some therapists tend to "explore the meaning" of cognitions and to focus on gaining insight into clients' "core schemas." DBT therapists, in contrast, use a linear model, assessing and analyzing all types of cognitions equally as they occur in the chain. When deciding which cognitions to treat, DBT therapists attend to factors such as their frequency and function and the degree to which they elicit dysfunctional affect or impulses.

CHAPTER 8

CONTINGENCY MANAGEMENT

KEY PRINCIPLES AND STRATEGIES

Contingency management procedures involve intentionally modifying behavior by "managing" the consequences of the behavior. Thus, the procedures require that therapists strategically utilize principles of normal learning processes to maximize clients' motivation to engage in skillful behavior and stop problematic behavior. Contingency management is a common component of parenting programs and, as discussed in Chapter 4, standard skills training involves shaping new skills with reinforcement. Of particular relevance to those who target substance abuse or dependence in their DBT programs, dismantling research (e.g., Carroll et al., 2006; Schumacher et al., 2007) has demonstrated that non-DBT drug treatment programs that include specific contingency management procedures have significantly better outcomes than programs without such procedures.

DBT applies contingency management when a BCA reveals that specific internal or external consequences of a client's behavior have reinforced a problematic behavior or have punished or extinguished skillful behavior. Reinforcement has occurred if the consequences of a behavior have increased the probability that the behavior will happen again. If a previously reinforced behavior has decreased because it no longer elicits the reinforcing consequences, then extinction has occurred. If a behavior has decreased because of the consequences that it elicits, then punishment has occurred. Therapists implement contingency management when they strategically change consequences to reinforce clients' skillful behaviors or to extinguish or even punish clients' target or other problematic behaviors. The sections below discuss each of these procedures in greater detail. Effective contingency management, however, often benefits from a combination of these procedures and multiple consequences within each procedure, as the case in Box 8.1 illustrates.

Contingency Managers

Involve Clients in Contingency Management

Whenever possible, therapists involve clients in changing the consequences of their behaviors. In some situations, clients can control the consequences themselves. In Jane's case, she and her therapist considered whether Jane could remove the reductions in guilt and shame as reinforcing consequences for vomiting (see Box 4.2 in Chapter 4). Jane achieved some success with this after her therapist taught her to challenge the beliefs that vomiting implied that she had gained control or punished herself. Many clients need to learn how and when to reward themselves for working toward a goal; otherwise they will extinguish the relevant behaviors because they think that rewards should occur only after achieving the goal completely or perfectly. Many clients also need to learn to stop punishing themselves for engaging in skillful behavior. For example, one client finally phoned for skills coaching instead of harming herself, but later in the week she harmed herself rather than phoned. In the next session she revealed that she had not phoned for coaching again because after the last coaching call she had berated herself for her performance on the phone and felt intense shame. She and her therapist then developed a plan to prevent these punishing consequences by replacing postcall performance analysis with mindful implementation of the coaching. They also added internal reinforcing consequences for seeking skills coaching (e.g., self-validation for completing the difficult task of phoning, mindfulness of gains resulting from call).

On other occasions, especially in interpersonal situations, clients cannot control all of the consequences of their behavior directly. In Rita's case, for example, the psychiatrist controlled when the session ended as much as Rita did, and the nurse entirely controlled whether and how she validated Rita. In such situations, however, clients may still implement contingency management by involving other relevant individuals as managers. In the case of Zelda, the client introduced in Chapter 6, her husband unintentionally reinforced her overdosing by becoming significantly more attentive and flattering following the overdoses. Though hesitant to implement any solution that could decrease her husband's attention, Zelda agreed that changing his response would extinguish her

Box 8.1. Contingency Management for Lola's Threatening

Near the end of a therapy session, Lola, an adult outpatient, suddenly began to threaten suicide. The therapist responded with a brief risk assessment, during which she adopted a more relational (e.g., using "we" and "us") and engaged style (e.g., leaning forward) than normal. When Lola's threats persisted, her therapist offered to extend the session to address the suicidal urges. She hypothesized that Lola might have anticipated feeling lonely after the session, as loneliness had led to the suicidal behavior that they had targeted during the session. Lola agreed with the hypothesis, and they proceeded to addressing the loneliness. Lola did not harm herself after the session, but again threatened suicide near the end of the next session. A brief risk assessment revealed although Lola had an elevated risk of self-harm, she was unlikely to kill herself. At this point, her therapist became more concerned about the reinforcement of threatening suicide than about Lola attempting suicide and hypothesized that the session extension had reinforced threatening. She referred Lola to the solutions that they had generated the previous week, but clarified that she would end the session on time. When Lola further escalated her threats, the therapist became more relational and soothing, but still ended on time.

The following week, the therapy targeted the last episode of threatening suicide. Though Lola had not threatened suicide with the intent of extending the session, the behavioral analysis, as well as her past learning history with mental health professionals, indicated that extending sessions had and would continue to reinforce suicidal threats, as such extensions allowed Lola to escape from the anticipated loneliness a while longer. The behavioral analysis also indicated that the therapist's increased relational and engaged style reinforced suicidal threats too, as the style decreased the client's general sense of isolation. As part of the solution analysis, Lola and her therapist agreed to attempt to extinguish the threatening by removing the identified reinforcing consequences. Furthermore, they identified alternative skillful behaviors that could achieve a function similar to the threatening but that the therapist could reinforce. Specifically, they decided to shape timely requests for help with and full participation in problem solving the anticipated loneliness. The therapist agreed that if Lola accomplished these behaviors and the therapist had extra time available, they would slightly extend the session. They also decided that the therapist could reinforce these behaviors by responding with an increase in her aforementioned relational and engaged style. They expected that the ultimate reinforcement for problem solving the loneliness would be, of course, less loneliness. Finally, they considered aversive consequences. They first differentiated threatening suicide from honestly reporting and directly requesting help for urges. They

(continued)

Box 8.1. (*continued*)

then agreed that if Lola threatened suicide, they would use the brief time remaining to conduct a risk assessment, and Lola consequently would lose the opportunity to problem solve the loneliness. Based on past experiences in Lola's treatment, they concluded that the threats might also decrease if the therapist responded to them in a confrontational or disengaged style. When Lola again threatened suicide at the end of the next session, her therapist implemented their plan. In subsequent sessions, Lola sometimes asked for help with the loneliness but she never again threatened suicide.

---

overdosing. As in Lola's case, Zelda and her therapist also identified more skillful behaviors that her husband could reinforce with increased attentiveness and flattery. Zelda then invited her husband to a session to discuss his potential role as a contingency manager. Susan's solution analyses for overdosing due to infidelity included changing consequences that either she or her boyfriend controlled. In the solution analysis (see Box 4.3 in Chapter 4), the therapist helped Susan to remove the reduction in guilt as a reinforcing consequence for overdosing by teaching her how to challenge the belief that she had absolved herself by overdosing and being hospitalized. In a later solution analysis, they tried to apply a similar set of strategies to remove the decrease in guilt and shame and increase in feeling connected to the boyfriend following his forgiveness. In-session rehearsal, however, revealed that this would not work. They decided to focus instead on changing how the boyfriend responded to the overdoses and invited him to a session to discuss possible changes. They decided that although the continuation of the relationship with the boyfriend required his forgiveness, the forgiveness needed to become contingent on Susan skillfully repairing the damage to the relationship and not at all associated with overdosing.

When involving clients in contingency management for the first time, therapists provide an orientation to the procedures, just as they would for any other solution. Therapists need to explain how consequences often shape behavior without the individual's awareness and to differentiate between conscious intent and reinforcing consequences of behavior, as illustrated by Susan's case. Making this distinction seems particularly important when a therapist suggests implementing contingency management to change interpersonal consequences that a client had not intended but that reinforced the target behavior. Lola initially objected when her therapist hypothesized that extending the session might have reinforced her threatening suicide at the end of the session. An analysis of this objection revealed that Lola thought that her therapist had implied that Lola "was trying to get" her therapist to extend the session and was "being manipulative." After her therapist explained how consequences rather than conscious intent can control behavior, Lola became notably more interested in identifying potential reinforcing consequences. Therapists might also need to address clients' judgmental or invalidating thoughts about the intentions and functions of behavior. For example, nonclinical and clinical environments alike have taught many clients to think of seeking attention as a "bad" or invalid thing to do. As Wilson and O'Leary (1980, p. 100) highlight, however, "social reinforcement in the form of adult attention and approval is probably the most powerful and versatile of all secondary [i.e., conditioned] reinforcers."

If the solution analysis involves another individual as contingency manager, clients first must orient that individual to contingency management and obtain the individual's commitment to implement the solution. Many clients decide to invite the individual to a therapy session or schedule an additional meeting together with the therapist, so that the therapist can assist them in the process. Susan and her therapist agreed to invite the boyfriend to a session primarily because they anticipated that otherwise Susan would avoid implementing the solution, as she wanted to avoid any discussions with her boyfriend about her infidelity. Zelda decided to invite her husband to a session because she had concerns that he would not "take it seriously" if she proposed it alone. Such meetings also give the therapist an opportunity to anticipate and address any potential problems with implementing contingency management. For example, many friends or family members fear that they will not be able to tolerate the client's escalating behavior if they try to extinguish it. Some feel guilty about the client's behavior and anticipate that this sense of guilt will interfere with implementing changes.

In some situations, clients choose to recruit another individual as a contingency manager without the client and that individual meeting with the therapist. For example, Mahly, a university student, identified how her mother's responses during telephone conversations punished several new emotion regulation and interpersonal skills (e.g., she interpreted her daughter's new ability to label emotions as an indicator of increasing emotionality). Her mother, however, could not attend a session because she lived across the country, and the treatment program did not have sufficient telecommunications facilities to bridge the gap. In Rita's case, she and her therapist could have met with the nurse whose validation reinforced the problematic behavior, but so many of the nurses responded the same way that inviting them all to therapy sessions would be impractical. In such situations, therapists consult with clients about how they can engage contingency managers by themselves. In Mahly's case, she and her therapist role-played how she could describe the new skills (e.g., labeling emotions) and their relevance (e.g., decreases emotionality) to her mother and ask her mother to reinforce the skills (e.g., validate daughter's hard work or progress, praise). The initial solution that Rita and her therapist generated for contingency problems with non-DBT inpatient staff required only minimal interpersonal skills to engage staff. With consultation from her therapist, Rita created a list of problematic and useful contingencies to enter in her file at the nurses' station. Successfully motivating other individuals to change the consequences that they control often requires that clients learn to validate those individuals' current responses first. After Rita's interpersonal skills had improved, her therapist decided that Rita could improve upon the lists in her file by speaking directly with the staff about their responses. When Rita and her therapist role-played how to do this, Rita competently described the conceptual aspects of contingencies as they related to her interactions with staff, but did so in a manner that would invalidate and irritate staff. Rita and her therapist then focused their role playing on this aspect of recruiting contingency managers. The emphasis in DBT on managing clients' interpersonal environments by consulting to clients rather than intervening for them (Linehan, 1993a) helps clients generalize the implementation of contingency management more broadly.

Sometimes individuals either cannot or will not implement contingency management procedures for clients' behaviors. In these situations, clients can still find ways to manage the contingencies. They might remain in the same environment with the same consequences, but change the salience of the consequences (e.g., with contingency clarification or stimulus control) or add more useful consequences. Mahly used both of these solutions. Though her discussions with her mother about contingencies had notably changed her mother's behavior, punishing responses remained. During conversations with her mother, Mahly minimized the salience of punishing responses by not attending too much to her mother's judgmental or otherwise invalidating comments. After these conversations, Mahly added reinforcing consequences by seeking validation from friends for having remained mindful, emotionally regulated, and interpersonally skillful while conversing with her mother. She also learned to praise herself for continuing to practice skills with her mother regardless of her mother's response. Clients who transition from living on welfare to starting low-paying jobs often lose more in benefits than they gain in salary. These clients might need to make the long-term financial gain more salient than the short-term loss or make social and psychological benefits more salient than financial ones. They might also need to structure additional immediate reinforcements (e.g., reward themselves with praise, obtain validation from family members, access social support at work). Some clients decide that they can "tolerate" problematic contingencies in one relationship if they spend more time in other relationships with reinforcing consequences for the same behavior. Therapists can help clients to identify and develop such environments. For example, one substance abusing client spent most of her time with her substance abusing husband, who had more motivation to continue reinforcing her drug use and extinguishing many of her new skills than he had to change his responses. The client did not want to leave her husband, so she and her therapist agreed that she would spend significantly more time in other existing relationships that reinforced skills use. She would also create opportunities to develop helpful new relationships through volunteering extensively in her church's charity activities. After the client began spending as much time in these contexts as she spent with her husband, the reinforcement that she received for skills use in those contexts helped to sustain her skills use with her husband.

Sometimes attempts at circumventing problematic contingencies do not suffice. In such situations clients might decide that they need to extricate themselves from the harmful relationship, develop more effective relationships, and seek their therapists' help to do so. Finally, if these attempts at circumventing problematic contingencies do not suffice, clients might decide that they need to extricate themselves from the harmful relationship, develop more effective relationships, and seek their therapists' help to do so. Max chose this option when he decided to end his relationships with his drug-dealing friends and seek friendships that reinforced his use of new skills.

Apply Contingency Management within DBT Treatment Context

In addition to assisting clients with managing contingencies in their natural environments, DBT clinicians manage contingencies within the DBT environment. DBT applies contingency management at both programmatic and individual levels. At the programmatic level, all clients in the program receive the same consequences for the same behaviors. For example, some skills training classes reward clients with a choice of small prizes for attending classes or completing homework. Similarly, some consultation teams reward members who arrive on time with refreshments. A few long-term inpatient and residential settings have extended this reward system to combine each patient's points into a grand total that counts toward a special event or treat for the class as a whole. Contingencies like this use social consequences to motivate collaborative behavior and inhibit nontherapeutic behavior. For example, a patient who tries to convince other patients to miss group with him or her might find fewer recruits with such a system, as everyone loses if anyone misses. Indeed, the client might meet with distinct disapproval from his or her peers. Some inpatient and residential settings require clients who engage in a behavior that in any way adversely affects the unit (e.g., self-harming in view of others, throwing furniture) to complete a repair protocol. Such protocols might include repairing whatever damage they have done to the best of their ability (e.g., publicly committing to implementing certain solutions to prevent self-harm, tidying the community areas for a period of time). It also might restrict clients' engagement in preferred activities (e.g., outings from the unit, chatting with nursing staff) until they have completed the protocol's requirements. Most standard outpatient DBT programs apply the "24-hour rule" (Linehan, 1993a) to telephone coaching, which removes clients' access to telephone coaching for 24 hours after any episode of self-harm. This program rule helps to break the contingency between suicidal behavior and greater access to clinicians, and to create a contingency between solving problems with skills and greater access to DBT therapists or skills coaches (Linehan & Heard, 1993). Finally, DBT programs change a key contingency that exists in many treatment contexts. Prior to starting DBT, many clients had the experience that stopping their most severe behaviors led therapists or other mental health professionals to reduce their availability, even though the clients still experienced internal distress. These clients learned that the only way to extend care was to maintain or return to the severe behaviors. DBT programs completely reverse this contingency by allowing clients to extend their initial DBT contract only if they have demonstrated a notable decrease in target behaviors and an increase in problem solving. Of course, not all consequences set by a program influence the behaviors of all clients, but programmatic contingencies do offer an efficient way to improve the motivation of most clients.

In most relationships, individuals respond to each other in ways that, intentionally or unintentionally, change the probability of each engaging in certain behaviors. Unfortunately, change can easily occur for the worse. Many clients, for example, have a history of receiving responses from therapists (e.g., extended session time, more sympathy or soothing, or decreased demands) as a consequence of target behaviors that stop the behavior in the short term, but inadvertently reinforce it in the long term. Individual therapists, therefore, acutely attend to how their responses influence each client and use this influence strategically to change all relevant client behaviors (e.g., suicidal and quality-of-life interfering behaviors, using skills daily), not just behaviors relevant to the treatment context (e.g., attending sessions, collaborating on analyses, completing homework, and phoning for coaching). Initially therapists may provide the only environment that alters contingencies to extinguish or punish a target behavior while simultaneously reinforcing more adaptive behaviors that can achieve the same function. In Lola's case, other care providers consistently and quickly reinforced her suicidal threats by responding with increased attention and thus decreased loneliness. Thus, her DBT therapist created the only environment that sufficiently motivated Lola to learn and implement new solutions for loneliness. For many clients, DBT clinicians provide the only sources of reinforcement for new skills, problem solving, or other critical but underused capabilities until the client has developed sufficient proficiency for these behaviors to elicit reinforcement from the external environment or to become internally reinforcing.

In-session client behaviors often provide the best opportunities for therapists to implement contingency management as they can immediately apply consequences. Lola's case, detailed in Box 8.1, illustrates the use of contingency management in treating an in-session behavior. Although some in-session behaviors may relate only to the therapy context (e.g., fully participating in skills rehearsal), most behaviors have relevance in multiple contexts (e.g., collaborating, independently noticing judgments, spontaneously generating solutions). Therapists use a variety of consequences in managing contingencies, including consequences related to the therapeutic relationship itself. Common reinforcing therapist responses include increasing validation, expressing more concern or interest, decreasing attempts to control the client, and offering to extend or shorten the session according to the client's wishes. Treating TIBs usually requires the withdrawal of reinforcement. For example, clients who want to avoid analyzing a specific behavior often impulsively repeat "I don't know" or "I can't remember" in response to therapists' questions, because they have learned in other contexts that such responses may stop additional questions and the analysis. In such cases, DBT therapists may successfully extinguish the behavior by persisting with the questions or otherwise continuing the analysis until the problematic behavior has stopped. Less frequently, therapists may use punishment.

For example, if a client finds the therapist's approval or attention desirable, the therapist might withdraw the approval or attention in response to noncollaborative behavior. When the client ceases the behavior and engages collaboratively again, the therapist then responds with approval or attention. Such a change in response by one individual to another's behavior more closely resembles the contingencies in relationships outside of therapy than would constant approval or attention. In one case, whenever the therapist rehearsed mindfulness with the client, the client would mindfully describe one thought and then immediately (and perhaps willfully) communicate a set of unmindful thoughts. After neither skills coaching during the session nor attempts at extinction had any obvious impact, the therapist began to assign additional mindfulness homework whenever the behavior occurred. After receiving only two or three additional assignments within the session, the client became motivated to remain mindful as long as possible.

The use of interpersonal consequences presents therapists with a small dilemma. On one side, therapists generally discuss contingency management options with clients, and clients (or at least some part of their brains) need to link their behavior with the consequence before the consequence can control the behavior. On the other side, interpersonal consequences often need to occur immediately to maximize their impact. Explaining the consequence can reduce the impact. For example, saying, "I'm now smiling at you and leaning forward to reinforce your collaboration" or "I'm now using a sharper tone and frowning to punish your refusal to rehearse this skill" may mean that the responses lose in impact what they gain in translation. Neither side of the dilemma is correct all of the time. Therapists generally seem to succeed if they respond in the most genuine way and then correct any misunderstandings that occur.

Assessment of Effective Consequences

Effective contingency management necessitates the assessment of new or changed consequences for their potency and availability in the environment. Therapists assess consequences both prior to and after their implementation. Reviews of previous analyses, attention to in-session interactions, and discussions with clients about reinforcing and punishing consequences each provide opportunities for assessment.

The potency of a consequence refers to the extent to which that consequence can control a specific behavior for a specific individual. Almost no consequence is a priori reinforcing or punishing for every individual, in every context, or for every behavior. Consequences receive the label of reinforcing or punishing only if they correspondingly increase or decrease the likelihood of the identified individual repeating the relevant behavior. The impact of a consequence for a designated behavior often varies significantly across individuals. For example, a look of disapproval from therapists will inhibit noncollaborative in-session behavior of some clients, whereas other clients note the look but only stop problematic behaviors if their therapists verbalize disapproval. Looks of disapproval are punishers of noncollaborative in-session behavior for the first client group, but not the latter.

The potency of a consequence depends on the form and dose (e.g., intensity, duration) of the consequence, as well as on the individual experiencing it. For example, humans generally experience validation from others as reinforcing (Swann et al., 1992), but the type of validation can affect whether it reinforces a behavior or not. In one case, a client increased practicing skills and implementing other solutions when his therapist responded by validating the difficulty of the task (Level 5 validation), but not when the therapist only listened to his report of implementation (Level 1 validation). Selecting potent consequences often requires specificity in defining the consequences. In Zelda's case, increased attentiveness from her husband meant looking at Zelda, talking with her, and otherwise interacting with her, not just spending time in the same room with her. In the case of an adolescent failing at school, praise from his parents or therapist for studying had no effect on studying, whereas praise from certain teachers did increase the studying. Another adolescent client experienced private praise from teachers as reinforcing, but public praise punishing. A consequence that controls one behavior might not control another behavior. In one case, praising the client's in-session behaviors increased those behaviors, but praising the client's homework completion had no impact on the likelihood of completion.

The availability of a consequence also determines its viability as part of a contingency management plan. For example, skills designed to decrease distress, aversive affect, and similar internal processes will have inherently reinforcing consequences after clients have developed proficiency, but clients may need more reliable sources of reinforcement, such as attention or approval from DBT clinicians, while still strengthening these skills. To maximize the likelihood of availability of consequences and the generalization of contingency management across contexts, therapists select natural over arbitrary consequences. Several DBT strategies involve responding to clients with natural contingencies, including being "radically genuine," as described in Chapter 1, and the "consistency agreement," described in Chapter 5. "Observing limits" (Linehan, 1993a) instructs therapists to apply contingency management when clients have crossed the therapists' natural personal limits. This contrasts with the approach in many treatments of setting limits based on arbitrary "boundaries." For example, DBT programs do not set limits as to when or how often clients can phone individual therapists for after-hours skills coaching. Instead, therapists inform clients about their own personal limits, which will more likely resemble the availability of important relationships in the clients' natural environments. If a client consistently crosses those limits, the therapist might respond with punishing consequences, such as reducing availability or describing the impact of the client's behavior on the therapist and therapeutic relationship. Such consequences frequently occur in clients' other relationships, though DBT therapists often articulate the contingencies more clearly. As part of preparing to end treatment, therapists and clients identify the contingencies in therapy that have contributed to clients' progress and, if they have not done so previously, work toward generalizing these contingencies to clients' other relevant environments to ensure that clients maintain their progress. For example, if validation from the therapist helped, the therapist and client might strengthen the clients' self-validation and teach a friend or family member about how and when to validate.

Reinforcement

Like most behavior therapies, DBT emphasizes reinforcement as the primary contingency management procedure. Therapists strategically increase clients' behaviors by directly applying reinforcing consequences within the therapy context (e.g., problem solving by a client who wants therapist involvement leads to a longer session with the therapist). They support clients' development of internally reinforcing behaviors, such as emotional regulation skills that reduce emotional pain and mindfulness skills that reduce cognitive suffering. They also help clients to elicit or arrange effective reinforcement in the natural environments (e.g., interpersonal skills lead to husband decreasing unwanted sexual demands, family agrees to allow an adolescent more freedom if he returns to school).

Identifying and implementing a variety of reinforcing consequences for any chosen behavior increases the likelihood of having consequences with sufficient availability and potency across a range of contexts. For example, if Lola's therapist did not have extra time available, she could still reinforce Lola's timely request for help by increasing relational statements in the moment. A reinforcing consequence can lose its effect and even become punitive if an individual becomes satiated. For example, paraphrasing what a client has said often reinforces clients for sharing information, but extensive paraphrasing can begin to sound like a little brother parroting his sister and become invalidating. To prevent satiation or its consequences, therapists and other contingency managers need a set of alternative reinforcing consequences.

The timing of reinforcement has a significant impact on its effectiveness. Immediate consequences have a significantly greater impact than delayed consequences. Similarly, intermittent or variable reinforcement minimizes the likelihood that a behavior will extinguish. As opposed to fixed schedules that require responding to a behavior after a specified interval or number of occurrences, variable schedules apply the consequence after unpredictable intervals or number of occurrences. Thus individuals do not know how long or how often they will need to engage in the behavior to obtain the desired response. In Lola's case, the unpredictable availability of the therapist increased the likelihood of Lola requesting problem-solving help rather than threatening. Though variable schedules prove the most resilient in the long term, contingency managers base the frequency of reinforcing consequences on the current strength of the behavior. Initially, contingency managers may reinforce clients each time they engage in the designated behavior and then move to a variable schedule. For example, the parents of an adolescent client failing at school initially rewarded each occasion of fully completing homework or passing an exam with a voucher for music (they did not need to worry about satiation). After the client began to regularly complete homework, they progressed to an increasingly variable reinforcement schedule.

Shaping refers to strengthening a behavior by reinforcing successive approximations to the desirable form, duration, or intensity of the behavior. When trying to shape a new or weak behavior, contingency managers may reward using separate components of the behavior or even just attempts at the behavior. For example, when teaching clients mindfulness, therapists might praise clients for just noticing judgments, even if the clients miss other types of problematic thoughts. Therapists might validate clients for rehearsing the components of the "DEAR MAN" skills, even if the style lacks grace or flow. Over time, however, therapists require increasing competency in the behavior to receive the same reward. For example, Chapter 5 describes the case of the therapist who required her client to have generated an increasing number of relevant skills before providing phone coaching. Rita's therapist initially provided some reinforcement for Rita's interpersonal skills practice as long as Rita had the correct form, but later required Rita to have a socially appropriate voice tone and body posture as well in order to receive the same reinforcement. If contingency managers demand too much before providing reinforcement, clients may become frustrated and stop engaging in the relevant behavior at all. Alternatively, if managers continue to provide the same level of reinforcement for the same level of behavior, clients may not develop sufficient competency for the behavior to become internally reinforcing or to obtain reinforcement in all relevant environments.

Extinction

Extinction procedures provide one option to decrease target and other problematic behaviors. As defined earlier, extinction procedures decrease a behavior by blocking reinforcing responses to the behavior. For example, one husband inadvertently reinforced his wife's cutting by bandaging her wounds, which decreased her sense of isolation from him. As part of the client's contingency management plan, the husband agreed that he would no longer bandage her wounds and would call a taxi for her if she needed medical treatment rather than accompanying her to the doctor's office. Lola's therapist implemented extinction when she stopped extending the therapy session in response to Lola's threats at the end of the session.

Whenever possible, therapists pair extinction of a target behavior with reinforcement and shaping of alternative behaviors that can achieve the same function as the target behavior. For example, spending less time during the homework review with clients who did not complete the homework reinforces some clients for not completing homework. In many classes, therefore, therapists do not focus less on clients who have not completed homework, but offer clients who have completed homework more choice about how much time they have for review and how they use that time. Susan and her therapist worked to extinguish overdosing by removing a key reinforcement for the behavior, namely reduction in guilt (see Box 4.3 in Chapter 4). Susan's tolerance of the extinction procedures depended, however, on the shaping of more skillful behaviors to manage the guilt and repair the damage to the relationship with her boyfriend. Similarly, Jane and her therapist used extinction to decrease vomiting by blocking decreases in guilt and shame through restructuring Jane's belief that vomiting meant that she had punished herself and exerted control (see Box 4.2 in Chapter 4). They paired the extinction with shaping skills to manage the emotions, repair "trouble" she had caused her mother, and gain effective control over her body. Identifying alternative behaviors allows contingency managers to implement differential reinforcement for situations that restrict the removal of reinforcing consequences for target behaviors. Differential reinforcement simply requires that the alternative behaviors receive more reinforcement than the target behavior. On one long-term DBT inpatient unit, close observation by nursing staff after suicidal behavior reinforced the suicidal behavior of a number of patients who wanted more attention from staff. Because of hospital policy and legitimate concerns about imminent risk, the staff could not stop providing observations. Instead, they arranged staffing on the unit to ensure that patients who requested skills coaching, assistance with solution implementation, or help with therapy tasks received even more attention. After implementing this program contingency, the staff noticed a significant decrease in suicidal behaviors.

During the course of extinction, clients sometimes experience escalations in the severity, intensity, duration, or frequency of target behaviors when the reinforcing consequence does not occur. Known as extinction or behavioral "bursts," these escalations can involve both overt behaviors (e.g., threatening suicide, yelling, threatening to write complaints) and covert behaviors (e.g., judging, experiencing auditory hallucination). Extinction bursts occur more often if the behavior has a history of variable reinforcement or if escalation itself has been rewarded. Identifying and reinforcing alternative behaviors can reduce the likelihood of such escalations. Behavioral bursts do not reduce the effectiveness of extinction procedures themselves, but if contingency managers then respond with reinforcement, they will have strengthened the original behavior *and* the escalation. To increase the likelihood of clients and other contingency managers tolerating an extinction burst, therapists provide information about the process and consultation about how to manage it. Susan and her therapist anticipated that if her boyfriend did not forgive her immediately, she might increase suicidal communications that he would have difficulty tolerating. The therapist coached the boyfriend on how to encourage Susan to repair instead of threatening overdoses, suggesting that he state that he expected to forgive Susan as soon as but not before she had repaired their relationship. The therapist also consulted with the boyfriend on how he could manage his own emotions. If the therapist, client, or wider environment cannot or will not tolerate a burst, then the solution analysis would not include withholding the reinforcing consequence.

Punishment

Punishment occurs in daily life, with or without intent, whenever aversive consequences of a behavior decrease the likelihood of the behavior occurring again. DBT therapists strategically and judiciously use this normal process to maximize the likelihood of quickly inhibiting severe target behaviors so that effective behaviors have the opportunity to strengthen. Contingency managers may implement punishment when a behavior needs to stop as quickly as possible because it presents an imminent danger to the client, other individuals, or the treatment. They also may implement punishment when they cannot control the reinforcing consequences of the behavior and either have no alternative behavior to reinforce or shaping other behaviors will require a prolonged period of work. For example, each time one client persistently disrupted a skills training class, the skills trainers asked the client to leave. The individual therapist knew that the dismissal reinforced the behavior by leading to decreased emotional arousal, but the skills trainers had to dismiss the client to preserve the class. Because the client also had a higher-order target, the therapist had little time to treat the disruptive behaviors by teaching the client how to manage the emotions leading to the behaviors. Therefore, the therapist included punishment as part of a short-term solution. The therapist expressed how the client's behavior impacted her motivation to work with the client and required that the client apologize to the class. She also clarified that if the behavior did not stop soon, she would suspend the treatment. These contingencies effectively decreased the disruptive behavior because the client valued her relationship and time with the therapist and hated having to apologize to the class. Though punishment tends only to suppress behavior in limited contexts and can produce negative side effects, contingency managers can minimize the side effects by applying punishment sparingly, not using it when they are highly emotional, providing the client with a rationale for the procedure, implementing punishment as the behavior begins, and reinforcing alternative behaviors (Wilson & O'Leary, 1980). As with reinforcement, immediate consequences punish behavior more effectively than delayed consequences, but in contrast to reinforcement, contingency managers need to implement punishing consequences consistently rather than intermittently.

A range of consequences can punish behavior. As with reinforcement, contingency managers often use social consequences to punish behavior. Many clients experience an expression of disapproval or confrontation as sufficiently aversive to stop behavior. Some clients experience a withdrawal of attention as punishing. With this type of client, a therapist might respond to the client's continued noncollaboration during a session by shortening the session. Losing the opportunity to do something pleasurable can inhibit a range of behaviors. For example, many therapists usually allow clients time to include topics besides target behaviors on the session agenda but remove this opportunity when clients engage in prolonged TIBs during the session.

"Correction–overcorrection" requires that clients not only correct their behavior or the damage done by their behavior, but that they overcorrect it by improving their behavior or repair the damage beyond normal requirements. The corrections should relate directly to the behavior or its natural effects. Furthermore, clients should not have access to other reinforcement in the same environment until they complete the overcorrection, at which time the punishment ends. For example, when one client screamed at her therapist in the therapy room and then turned over a table and broke a vase in reception, her therapist phoned her to say that she could not return to the clinic or access after-hours phone coaching until she had repaired the damage that she had done. Also, she could contact her therapist during working hours only to seek coaching on how to implement correction–overcorrection. The therapist specifically required the client to complete a detailed BCA and solution analysis for the set of behaviors (not a standard requirement for the client), implement or at least rehearse the solutions, apologize "beyond expectation" to the receptionist and the therapist, and replace the vase. When the client arrived at her session the following week, she had completed the analysis and at least rehearsed most of the solutions. She had apologized to the therapist verbally and with a card and to the receptionist with a card and a bouquet of flowers (she had consulted with the therapist about this). The replacement vase did not quite coordinate with the reception area, but could serve other uses in the clinic. At this time, the therapist welcomed her to their session.

If none of these consequences, as part of a comprehensive solution analysis, sufficiently inhibit an extreme target behavior, therapists may consider suspending treatment completely for an extended period of time. Suspensions usually involve not only a set amount of time but also completing designated tasks or solving specified problems. Therapists use such suspensions rarely and usually only after an extreme behavior that exceeds the therapist's or program's limits (e.g., physically assaulting the therapist, threatening other clients) or after prolonged efforts to change the behavior with thorough solution analyses.

COMMON PROBLEMS

Issues Impacting All Procedures

Foremost among the problems that occur are therapists neglecting contingency management procedures altogether in the solution analysis. Other therapists attempt to include the procedures but remain confused about the basic concept of contingencies. Therapists who have a basic understanding of the procedures and use them may still make errors in their assessment and selection of effective consequences. These include making assumptions about the potency of consequences and not specifying consequences sufficiently. When applying extinction or punishment, contingency managers sometimes implement the procedures inconsistently or forget to balance them with reinforcement of alternative skillful behaviors. Though intermittent reinforcement strengthens behavior more than fixed reinforcement does, inconsistent punishment or extinction will reduce the effectiveness of the procedures and possibly lead to more harm than improvement. Finally, therapists may reduce the impact of contingency management if they do not attend to the availability and generalization of the consequences.

Neglecting Contingency Management

As with other CBT solutions, therapists sometimes reduce the effectiveness of a solution analysis by neglecting to include contingency managing procedures. Such neglect occasionally occurs because the therapist believes that clients should learn to control behavior through self-regulation rather than with external environmental consequences. For example, in one forensic setting, a therapist dismissed contingency management procedures because he believed that behavior changes resulting from environmental consequences rather than clients' "internal motivation" were "insincere" and "could not last." The team initially tried to treat the belief with cognitive restructuring (e.g., reviewing empirical evidence in the literature, suggesting that the therapist perform experiments) and mindfulness (noticing the belief and then refocusing his attention on delivering the treatment adherently). When neither of these standard solutions worked, the team applied contingency management to the therapist. They reminded him that he had made a commitment to apply the treatment as adherently as possible and stated that if he persisted in breaking his commitment, they would have to reconsider his membership with the team. More often therapists neglect contingency management because they do not know when to use it, how to apply it, or both. This pair of problems can be addressed with didactic teaching. Consultation teams can review solution analyses to identify and correct therapist lack of awareness and conduct role plays to model and shape the application of contingency management procedures.

Misunderstanding Contingent Relationships

Most therapists who have no previous training in behaviorism or contingency management initially struggle with describing contingent relationships. In behavioral therapies, contingent relationship refers to the relationship between a behavior and a consequence in which the consequence occurs only following the behavior. Thus, describing contingent relationships requires identifying a behavior and a consequence. Many therapists without behavioral training, however, identify consequences without identifying corresponding behaviors. For example, a therapist may identify "praise" as a reinforcer used for contingency management but not identify the client's behavior(s) upon which praise is contingent. A conceptually clearer description might be "praise reinforces in-session skills rehearsal and out-of-session homework completion." Some therapists make the error of identifying antecedent–behavior links instead of behavior–consequence links as relevant contingent relationships. For example, "reminding client of homework assignments" is an antecedent rather than a consequence of homework completion. Adding reminders as a solution, therefore, would be stimulus control rather than contingency management. Therapists can correct these conceptual errors if they think of contingent relationships as requiring two columns: one identifies the behavior to increase or decrease and the other identifies consequences that increase or decrease that behavior.

Making Assumptions about the Potency of Consequences

Some therapists and other contingency managers make automatic assumptions about the potency of consequences. This occurs most often when contingency managers confuse the scientific definitions of reinforcement and punishment with a lay definition that considers certain consequences as reinforcing or punishing a priori. A frequent indicator that a contingency manager has made an automatic assumption about consequences is if he or she says, "Punishment doesn't work for this client because the behavior didn't decrease when I tried it" (or the opposite for reinforcement). A consequence is punishing only if it decreases the designated behavior and reinforcing only if it increases the behavior. For example, many people assume that everyone experiences praise as reinforcing. Research, however, has revealed that depressed clients are not rewarded by positive statements from others that contradict their own negative beliefs about themselves (e.g., Swann et al., 1992). Therapists working with BPD clients often have found that praise actually punishes clients for reducing target behaviors. Many of these clients had previous treatment in which praise of progress became associated with service withdrawal or life experiences in which praise became associated with increased demands or responsibilities (e.g., resuming child care duties, returning to work). Contingency managers need to check with clients and not assume what will be reinforcing to them.

Not Specifying Consequences Sufficiently

Therapists sometimes do not specify a consequence sufficiently and thus reduce the potency of the consequence or miss an opportunity to implement it. For example, when clients' behaviors have harmed others, many therapists have instructed clients to "repair" as part of correction–overcorrection, but have not consulted with the clients about how to repair. In such instances, many clients then simply apologize to the other person. Apologies, however, often do not repair the actual damage that the client caused and almost never overcorrect the damage. For example, when one client's disruptive behavior in skills class distressed other clients in the class and caused a loss in teaching time, her therapist requested that she "repair to the group." The skills trainers reported to the therapist that the client had apologized to the group, but stated that this had not actually repaired the damage. Implementing repair as a correction–overcorrection technique usually necessitates that the therapist and client identify the actual damage and how the client can repair that damage, plus a little extra. In the case above, when the client again disrupted the skills class, her therapist taught her how to match damage and repairs. For the lost learning time, they decided that the client would search the Internet for additional materials related to the teaching topic of the week and bring copies of this material to class for everyone. To address the distress she had caused, she decided to bring a soothing lavender-scented candle and herbal teas.

In another case, the therapist initially missed an opportunity to extinguish the suicidal behavior of Marian, an inpatient, because he did not specify the consequences sufficiently. He knew from behavioral analyses that being placed on observations following suicidal behavior reinforced the behavior. He briefly considered extinction, but knew that the inpatient staff could not reduce observations as a response because of unit policy. He tried to change the relevant contingencies by encouraging the staff to increase their responses to the client's problem-solving behaviors, but the client's suicidal behavior persisted. When he reviewed his solution analysis with the team, they suggested that he might be able to include extinction if he considered whether the unit could withdraw any of the specific consequences associated with observations. The therapist then identified that although the staff would have to remain within physical proximity to the client, they could stop chatting with the client and trying to reassure or soothe her, all of which reinforced the suicidal behavior more than someone simply watching.

Inconsistently Applying Punishment or Extinction

Contingency managers sometimes identify specific, potent consequences to reduce a behavior, but then do not implement the consequences consistently. Applying aversive consequences intermittently tends to reduce the likelihood that the consequences will punish behavior. Inconsistency seems to appear most often when the consequence depends on multiple contingency managers (e.g., extensive non-DBT outpatient treatment team, inpatient unit, multiple family members) or when individual contingency managers, including therapists, vary in their own capacity or motivation (e.g., available time or energy, emotional state) to implement the procedures. For example, in one family the father implemented contingency procedures more consistently than the mother, though he spent less time with the client and had less opportunity to shape the behavior. The mother's application varied significantly, with notable lapses in the morning when she had to rush to her job and in the evening when she felt tired. Consultation teams can help therapists and therapists can help other contingency managers to treat the variables than control inconsistency, but if the inconsistency persists, the therapist may decide to remove the relevant contingency management procedures from the solution analysis.

Not Balancing Extinction and Punishment with Reinforcement

Contingency managers increase the probability of side effects from extinction and punishment procedures if they do not pair those procedures with encouraging or reinforcing alternative, adaptive behaviors that achieve the same function as the problematic behavior. When therapists fail to balance decreasing a target behavior with increasing skillful behaviors, clients often substitute one target behavior for another. For example, one residential unit with a DBT program successfully extinguished suicidal threats by no longer transferring a client onto the less demanding acute ward following threats. The client, however, started reporting more frequent and severe hallucinations, which also prompted transfers to the acute unit. The therapist realized that during consultations with the client and unit staff, she had focused on how to stop reinforcing the threats and had neglected to identify alternative behaviors that the client could use to modify or tolerate demands and that the staff could then reinforce. An absence of attention to alternative behaviors during extinction also increases the likelihood of a behavioral burst. For example, the staff on an inpatient unit had agreed not to solve a client's problems for her (e.g., resolving interpersonal conflict) following episodes of cutting, as analyses had indicated that such a consequence reinforced the cutting. Unfortunately, while trying to extinguish the cutting, it escalated. Though the escalations seemed like temporary extinction bursts, the therapist thought that if the bursts continued, the staff would either forgo extinction or reinforce the bursts. In reviewing the extinction implementation, the therapist realized that he had not attended enough to how the staff could coach the client to solve her own problems and reinforce her for doing so. Contingency managers who apply punishment without offering opportunities to obtain desired consequences through other behaviors risk alienating or at least damaging their relationships with clients.

Not Attending to Generalization of Consequences

Clients may improve during treatment, but then deteriorate after treatment because their therapists have not attended to the availability and generalization of useful contingencies. This seems to occur particularly in systems that reinforce behaviors above the levels available in clients' daily lives or that rely on potent aversive consequences to inhibit behavior. For example, some patients have difficulty transitioning from inpatient units to outpatient settings because they no longer have such frequent environmental reinforcement for the behaviors needed to maintain their progress. Clients in court-ordered treatment programs often suppress target behaviors during the program to avoid the punishment that the program would impose, but then return to the behavior after the program and its consequences end. Therapists can attempt to increase the generalization of consequences in several ways. For example, they can identify the useful contingencies in treatment and then teach the client how to arrange more useful consequences in the environment or consult with the client and the environment together. Many include this as a standard task during the ending phase of treatment. If a consequence commonly used to motivate behavior in the natural environment has a minimal (or even opposite) effect on a client, the therapist can attempt to recondition the client's response to that consequence over time. For example, if praise of behaviors leading to progress punished those behaviors, the therapist could initially use other consequences (e.g., validation, extra session time, decrease of demands) to reinforce the behaviors and then start to pair those reinforcing consequences with praise. As long as the praise did not coincide with aversive consequences again, it could develop into a reinforcing consequence itself. In several cases, therapists have helped clients with antisocial behaviors to develop new value systems such that the clients essentially punish any reoccurrences of antisocial behavior themselves. Finally, decreasing reinforcement within the treatment setting over time to a level below whatever the natural environment offers can facilitate the transition for some clients.

Extinction

Reinforcing Target Behaviors

In many cases, therapists or other contingency managers continue to reinforce target behaviors when extinction could prove useful. In some instances, therapists may not have considered extinction because they failed to identify the reinforcing consequence during a behavioral analysis. For example, many therapists complain to their consultation teams when clients distract from analyses during sessions with other topics or prolonged narratives, but frequently these therapists lack an awareness of how listening to clients distract reinforces the distracting. Consultation teams can help to identify such opportunities for extinction through reviews of therapists' solution analyses or session recordings. On other occasions, therapists have identified an opportunity to use extinction but the relevant contingency mangers have skills or motivational deficits that prevent implementation. With an analysis of the variables preventing the implementation of extinction, consultation teams or therapists can generate appropriate solutions. For example, a therapist reported that she knew that her listening reinforced her client distracting to other topics, but she thought that interrupting "would be rude" and feared that the client would become angry. Irreverent cognitive restructuring from the team addressed the cognition. The team then role played with the therapist how to interrupt in a way that would minimize anger and how to manage any angry response. Less often, therapists exclude extinction because of inaccurate assumptions about the practical viability of the procedure, as described in Marian's case above.

At the program level, the most significant problem occurs when programs extend therapy contracts for clients who have deteriorated or demonstrated no notable progress during the course of treatment. In such programs, clients often learn that the best way to secure more treatment is to maintain severe target behaviors. Adherent DBT programs avoid this problem by reversing the contingency. Only clients who have demonstrated some benefit from the treatment receive offers of more DBT treatment.

Reinforcing Behavioral Bursts

Contingency managers sometimes strengthen the behavior they want to weaken by beginning extinction procedures and then reinforcing an extinction burst. Of course, if the behavior escalates to the extent that it threatens someone's life, then saving the life takes priority. On other occasions, however, managers stop the extinction in response to the extinction burst but without any risk assessment or obvious risk. This usually occurs because the managers either have mistakenly interpreted the burst as an indication that the extinction procedures have not worked or have become too distressed themselves. Providing training about the process of extinction can reduce inaccurate assumptions. Additional training in the relevant risk assessments may help managers, especially therapists, to discern when a burst does not warrant fear and thereby decrease the frequency of unjustified fear. To address the distress and any unwarranted emotions, consultation teams or therapists can assess whether any variables other than the burst itself control the emotional distress and generate solutions accordingly.

Punishment
Excluding Punishment for Nonclinical Reasons

A few therapists include reinforcement and extinction in solution analyses, but automatically exclude punishment procedures. This occurs most often when therapists misunderstand the concept of punishment, have inaccurate information about its effectiveness, are judgmental about using it, or have an emotional response. The most common misunderstandings include confusing the scientific definition with lay uses of the term such as to be punitive (i.e., to treat harshly or attempt to inflict suffering). Frequent judgments include "Therapist's shouldn't use punishment," "It's unethical," "It's mean," I'm being mean," and "I'm being unkind." Possible solutions that consultation teams can use for problematic cognitions include presenting the scientific definition of punishment and empirical research on it, highlighting ways in which the therapist already punishes behaviors without awareness or intent, reviewing the pros and cons of punishment, and helping the therapist to become mindful of judgmental thinking. Common emotional inhibitors include fear and guilt. Assuming that the context justifies neither of these emotions, the consultation team might treat the emotions with either skills or exposure. In one case, a therapist reported that both judgmental thoughts of "I'm being mean" and guilt inhibited her from applying potentially effective punishment in the form of expressing disapproval. In this instance the therapist found cognitive restructuring and mindfulness both helpful for the judgmental thought, but emotion regulation skills and mindfulness did not have the expected impact on the guilt. A more detailed discussion revealed that in previous attempts at punishment with other clients, the distressed look on clients' faces following expressions of disapproval had prompted the guilt. The team then decided to try exposure. During the consultation meeting, the therapist role played expressing disapproval to "clients" while they expressed great distress in their faces. After the consultation meeting, the therapist imagined the same scenario with her clients. The exposure proved more effective than the emotion regulation skills had.

Overutilizing Aversive Consequences

A more severe problem related to punishment involves overutilizing aversive consequences to control behavior. The problem includes applying punishment too frequently or severely (i.e., the punishment does not fit the crime) and becoming punitive rather than punishing. Research has suggested that staff with limited training in DBT might engage in such behaviors more frequently than staff with advanced training (Trupin, Stewart, Beach, & Boesky, 2002). These behaviors also appear more likely among nonclinical contingency managers such as parents and in involuntary institutions such as court-ordered outpatient drug treatment programs, forensic inpatient units, and prisons. Trupin et al.'s (2002) study indicates that more training in contingency management may reduce the problem, though therapists and clients involving nonclinical individuals as contingency managers may need to continue to monitor and consult with those managers regularly. Regardless of training or institution, all contingency managers, including therapists, remain vulnerable to overutilizing aversive consequences when clients' behaviors elicit strong emotions in the contingency manager. To prevent or correct any therapist who engages in such behavior, consultation teams balance problem solving and other change strategies with validation and other acceptance strategies. Therapists also offer similar consultation to non-DBT contingency managers. For example, when the mother of one adolescent client initially seemed more punitive than strategically punishing, the therapist reviewed the principles of contingency management and helped the mother and daughter to identify specific punishing consequences of a useful potency for specific behaviors. Though the mother implemented the contingencies that they had discussed, she continued to respond in a punitive manner. Through a more detailed analysis with the mother, the therapist discovered that the more punitive behaviors occurred only if the mother had become very angry about her daughter's behavior. The therapist both validated the mother's anger and coached her on how to implement a combination of anger management skills that the mother had learned in the skills training class, which she attended with her daughter.

EPILOGUE

PROBLEM-SOLVING THERAPISTS' BEHAVIORS

An Illustration

Although the book has included many examples of how therapists and consultation teams have applied problem-solving strategies to treat therapists' problematic behaviors, it has not presented a complete analysis of any therapist behavior. DBT, however, strongly emphasizes the importance of treating therapist behaviors as well as client behaviors and assigns an entire modality for this purpose. Therefore, it seemed fitting to end the book with a more detailed illustration of how a consultation team might treat the problematic behavior of one of its members.

Although in most instances, teams only have enough time to review or conduct a brief, informal analysis of the factors controlling a therapist's behavior and to generate and implement only one or two solutions, they sometimes decide to complete lengthier, formal behavioral chain and solution analysis. The team may need to conduct a structured, comprehensive analysis because the severity of the behavior or the complexity of the factors controlling it warrants such an analysis. The team may also choose to use a portion of their teaching time for this type of analysis as a way to enhance their competency in applying these strategies with clients. These more substantial analyses usually progress more efficiently and effectively if one team member takes responsibility for structuring and guiding the analysis and preventing the identified therapist from becoming overwhelmed with questions, opinions, or even reassurance from others. This process also requires willingness on the part of the identified therapist, of course, though no more than therapists require from clients every week. These comprehensive analyses can benefit the team by directly reducing the problematic behavior of the identified therapist, indirectly reducing similar behaviors by other members, and improving everyone's knowledge of DBT and competency in implementing it.

This illustration involves Alice, a therapist who recently joined a DBT program for adolescents who would meet criteria for BPD except for their age. Prior to entering treatment, Alice's client had made multiple suicide attempts, but these rapidly decreased following the introduction of emotion regulation skills. Only after 3 months in treatment, however, did Alice become aware that her client also met criteria for anorexia, as the client had lied about this behavior during the pretreatment assessment. About a month after this revelation, Alice arrived 30 minutes late to the consultation team, explaining that she had had to meet with her client and the client's parents. At the end of the meeting, the consultation team requested that Alice bring a written BCA of missing 30 minutes to review during the next consultation meeting. They decided to use the teaching portion of the consultation meeting so that they would have sufficient time both to address Alice's behavior and to teach newer therapists more about key problem-solving principles and strategies.

Alice brought the BCA illustrated in Box E.1. She specified the target behavior clearly as "offering to extend the therapy session into the consultation meeting time." The team then noted that Alice had described the function of offering as "reduces aversive emotions," but had not specified which emotions. Though she could have intended the statement as a summary for anxiety, shame, and anger, the details of the analysis also suggest that the different emotions may have played different roles as controlling variables. Further hypothesizing and analysis suggested that the offer to extend the session functioned primarily to decrease Alice's anxiety, though Alice thought that the reduction in shame might have provided additional reinforcement. Alice decided that the reduction in anger would not reinforce the target behavior. Instead, she agreed with the team's hypothesis that the anger had functioned to decrease the anxiety and fear and to "give her permission" to miss the consultation team. Based on the target behavior's functions, Alice and the team decided to focus the solution analysis first on links related to the anxiety and "helping the family." If time permitted, they would then progress to the other emotions and other consequences of her behavior. The team also clarified that the client's BMI dropping to 18 and the family arriving 20 minutes late for the session were vulnerability factors

---

Box E.1. BCA and Solution Analysis
for Missing a Consultation Meeting

Target: Offers to extend therapy session into consultation meeting time.

Function of the target: Reduce therapist anxiety and increase therapist's thoughts of being helpful to the family.

Links	Generated Solutions
Client's BMI has dropped to 18.	
Parents and client arrived 20 minutes late for joint session.	
Client expressed anger about elements of the solution analysis and refused to implement it.	**Conduct a brief BCA on the refusal and treat key links.**
Anxiety (2/5).	**Mindfulness of emotion, radical acceptance.**
Thinks, "This treatment is not going well."	**Mindful description, dialectical thinking.**
Thinks, "She will end up in the hospital."	Examining the evidence, **mindfulness of present task.**
Anxiety increases (3/5).	Mindfulness of emotion.
Notices only 10 minutes remaining before consultation team.	
Thinks, "I really need to get her commitment now."	
Anxiety increases (4/5).	**Act opposite to tensing body.**
Thinks, "I'm no good with anorexics."	
Shame (3/5).	
Thinks, "Don't be ridiculous. She just doesn't understand what will happen if she doesn't change. I just need to help her see the importance of these solutions."	**Mindfulness of assumption.**
Reviews with the client reasons to use solutions.	**Conduct a brief BCA on the refusal and assign homework to treat key links.**
Client continues to refuse to implement solutions.	
Notices only 5 minutes remaining.	
Anxiety increases (5/5).	**Act opposite to tensing body.**
Thinks, "I could extend the session for half an hour."	**Contingency clarification**

(continued)

Box E.1. (*continued*)

Anxiety decreases (4/5).

Urge to extend session (3/5).   **Act opposite by starting to end session.**

Thinks, "This is more important than a   **Contingency clarification.**
  team meeting."

Thinks, "The team should understand."

Anger (2/5).

Thinks, "I shouldn't have to have such
  a booked caseload. What can people
  expect?"

Anger increases (4/5).

Anxiety decreases (3/5), shame decreases
  (2/5).

Thinks, "I'm just going to take my time."

Offers to extend session time.   **Act opposite by ending session.**

Anxiety decreases (1/5).

Mother says that she really appreciates
  the help.

Shame and anger disappear.

Thinks, "I am a really responsive, helpful   Dialectical thinking.
  therapist."

Returns to attempting to increase the
  client's motivation to implement solutions.

Client agrees to implement solutions.

Arrives 30 minutes late to consultation team.

Team warmly welcomes me.   **Contingency management.**

At the end of the meeting, the team requests
  that I bring a written BCA of missing 30
  minutes to the next meeting.

Writes BCA.

Anxiety (2/5) about reviewing BCA.

Note. **Bold font = solutions implemented**; standard font = solutions generated only.

---

rather than links in the chain. They agreed not to address these links as the client seldom arrived late, and it would require the entire treatment to change the behaviors that decreased the BMI.

With respect to treating the anxiety itself, Alice and the team generated more acceptance-based skills for lower levels of anxiety and more change-based skills for higher levels. Alice thought that simple mindfulness of the emotion would work if the emotion remained at an intensity of 2 but doubted that mindfulness would suffice if it escalated to a 3. She rehearsed the team's suggestion of radically accepting some degree of emotion when working with this client population and anticipated that the skill would work at 2, a level that she thought the situation justified, but not beyond this level. Once the emotion had escalated to a 4, Alice had become aware of assuming a tense body posture and slightly clenching her hands. The team discussed how Alice could act opposite to tensing without stopping the therapy session. After trying a couple of ideas, Alice found it most useful to stretch her back and hands subtly and then lean her back against the chair and rest her hands flat in her lap. The most significant action urge associated with the anxiety was offering to extend the session. For this, the team suggested not just inhibiting the urge but acting opposite to the urge, namely, highlighting to the family that the session would soon end and then implementing session-ending strategies (e.g., summarizing session, identifying or reviewing homework assignments, planning for the next session). Alice and the team then role played and shaped these strategies, with additional attention to body posture.

As Alice's initial cognitions seemed to escalate her anxiety as much as the client's refusal did, the team also identified cognitions to treat. For the thought "This treatment is not going well," the therapist rehearsed mindfully describing the actual problem in the session (e.g., "The client has refused to implement the solutions") rather than overgeneralizing. This mindful description both helped prevent the anxiety from escalating and better prepared Alice to target the client's refusal. The team also suggested thinking more dialectically about the treatment. Though Alice thought that this could decrease her anxiety, she thought that it might require too much time during a session, but she agreed to practice it more between sessions. For "She will end up in the hospital," Alice thought that mindfully returning her attention to the present moment and task would help, but she did not think that examining the evidence for this belief would help, as reviewing the evidence would also take time, and any evidence to support her belief would increase her anxiety. She anticipated that as her emotions increased, her ability to use mindfulness would decrease. The team did highlight, however, that her automatic assumptions about what controlled the client's behavior (i.e., "She just doesn't understand . . .") caused her to choose cognitive solutions (i.e., reviewing with the client reasons to use solutions) without first understanding why the client had refused. The assumption proved inaccurate and thus contributed to the client's second refusal. The team encouraged the therapist to become more mindful of such assumptions as part of her general clinical development.

Alice's later cognitions did not increase her anxiety, but seemed to function to "give permission" to miss the consultation team meeting. For these thoughts, the team primarily used contingency clarification. In particular, they highlighted that Alice had correctly recognized that she had no expertise in treating anorexia and then chose to miss the one meeting that could help her gain the expertise that she needed. They also described how one member choosing to miss part of a consultation meeting can decrease the motivation of the entire team to arrive on time. The team also reminded Alice that the meeting functioned as therapy for the therapists and asked whether she would have extended the therapy session with her client if she had had a skills class scheduled next rather than the consultation meeting. The use of contingency clarification significantly shifted Alice's thoughts about the importance of the consultation meeting and extending therapy sessions into consultation meetings.

As the extension of the session also functioned to help the client, the team discussed how Alice could have helped the client more during the initial 30 minutes, as well as how to accept that she may not achieve everything that she wants to achieve in any given session. The team particularly encouraged Alice to conduct a brief BCA on the client's refusal to implement solutions. The team thought that after the first refusal Alice would still have time to implement solutions as well, but after the second refusal she would only have time to generate some solutions and assign relevant homework. Alice and the team then rehearsed these two scenarios with role plays.

Finally, the team reviewed how well they had managed contingencies following Alice's arrival. They had followed through with the standard procedure of requesting a BCA and then conducting a solution analysis for unauthorized absences. Though these analyses served primarily as the means to identify and treat key controlling variables, in Alice's case they also punished the target behavior, as the written BCA cost time and the review during the consultation team meeting cost emotionally. The team commended Alice on noticing their warm welcome and wondered whether they should respond differently to team members who arrive late. They considered, however, whether a neutral response to late arrivals might discourage them from arriving at all that week. They also doubted that a warm welcome would reinforce anyone's tardiness. They agreed that they would aim to welcome late arrivals, but not as warmly as those who arrived on time.

Following this analysis, Alice did not repeat her target behavior. She also reported that her ability to target clients' in-session behaviors had improved. She attributed this to having become more competent at mindfully describing a client's in-session behavior, identifying her assumptions about the behavior as assumptions, and then conducting a brief BCA on the client's behavior. She still had some difficulty in generating solutions following the brief BCA, but sought more solutions from the team. Finally, Alice reported tolerating warranted levels of anxiety better and using cognitive solutions, especially mindfulness, to prevent the anxiety from escalating.

Alice's case demonstrates how DBT uses the same behavioral conceptualization and problem-solving strategies to treat therapists' interfering behaviors and clients' target behaviors. The team first behaviorally defined a target for analysis. Alice completed her own BCA in which she identified controlling variables for the target. She especially attended to her emotions throughout the chain. The team and Alice then clarified the target behavior's function and focused their solution analysis on addressing this function. They generated a variety of CBT procedures as solutions, including skills, cognitive restructuring, and contingency management, and attended to balancing change-based procedures with acceptance-based skills. Their solution analysis also included solution evaluation and implementation. For example, Alice rehearsed weaker skills and then the team shaped these skills through coaching. For Alice, completing and reviewing the BCA was an important part of implementing contingency management. Applying the same behavioral conceptualization and strategies to therapists and clients alike exemplifies how the principles of learning and changing behavior used in DBT are not just for individuals with psychological problems but instead are universal.

REFERENCES

Abramowitz, J. S., Deacon, B. J., & Whiteside, S. P. H. (2010). *Exposure therapy for anxiety: Principles and practice.* New York: Guilford Press.

Aitken, R. (1982). *Taking the path of Zen.* San Francisco: North Point.

American Psychiatric Association. (1994). *Diagnostic and statistical manual of mental disorders* (4th ed.). Washington, DC: Author.

American Psychiatric Association. (2013). *Diagnostic and statistical manual of mental disorders* (5th ed.). Arlington, VA: Author.

Anderson, C. A. (1989). Temperature and aggression: Ubiquitous effects of heat on occurrence of human violence. *Psychological Bulletin, 106,* 74–96.

Bandura, A. (1971). Psychotherapy based on modeling principles. In A. E. Bergin & S. L. Garfield (Eds.), *Handbook of psychotherapy and behavior change* (pp. 653–708). New York: Wiley.

Bantick, S. J., Wise, R. G., Ploghaus, A., Clare, S., Smith, S. M., & Tracey, I. (2002). Imaging how attention modulates pain in humans using functional MRI. *Brain, 125,* 310–319.

Bar-Haim, Y., Lamy, D., Pergamin, L., Bakermans-Kranenburg, M. J., & van IJzendoorn, M. H. (2007). Threat-related attentional bias in anxious and non-anxious individuals: A meta-analytic study. *Psychological Bulletin, 133,* 1–24.

Barlow, D. H. (2002). *Anxiety and its disorders: The nature and treatment of anxiety and panic* (2nd ed.). New York: Guilford Press.

Barrett, L. F., Gross, J., Christensen, T. C., & Benvenuto, M. (2001). Knowing what you're feeling and knowing what to do about it: Mapping the relation between emotion differentiation and emotion regulation. *Cognition and Emotion, 15,* 713–724.

Basseches, M. (1984). *Dialectical thinking and adult development.* Norwood, NJ: Ablex.

Beck, A. T., Rush, A. J., Shaw, B. F., & Emery, G. (1979). *Cognitive therapy of depression.* New York: Guilford Press.

Beck, A. T., & Weishaar, M. E. (1989). Cognitive therapy. In R. J. Corsini

& D. Wedding (Eds.), *Current psychotherapies* (pp. 285–323). Itasca, IL: Peacock.

Bijttebier, P., & Vertommen, H. (1999). Coping strategies in relation to personality disorders. *Personality and Individual Differences, 26*, 847–856.

Bonanno, G. A., Papa, A., Lalande, K., Westphal, M., & Coifman, K. (2004). The importance of being flexible: The ability to both enhance and suppress emotional expression predicts long-term adjustment. *Psychological Science, 15*, 482–487.

Bryant, R. A., Kenny, L., Joscelyne, A., Rawson, N., Maccallum, F., Cahill, C., et al. (2014). Treating prolonged grief disorder: A randomized clinical trial. *JAMA Psychiatry, 71*, 1332–1339.

Carroll, K. M., Easton, C. J., Nich, C., Hunkele, K. A., Neavins, T. M., Sinha, R., et al. (2006). The use of contingency management and motivational/skills-building therapy to treat young adults with marijuana dependence. *Journal of Consulting and Clinical Psychology, 74*, 955–966.

Corsini, R. J., & Wedding, D. (1989). *Current psychotherapies*. Itasca, IL: Peacock.

Demiralp, E., Thompson, R. J., Mata, J., Jaeggi, S. M., Buschkuehl, M., Feldman Barrett, L., et al. (2012). Feeling blue or turquoise?: Emotional differentiation in major depressive disorder. *Psychological Science, 23*, 1410–1416.

D'Zurilla, T. J., & Goldfried, M. R. (1971). Problem solving and behavior modification. *Journal of Abnormal Psychology, 78*, 107–126.

D'Zurilla, T. J., & Nezu, A. M. (1999). *Problem-solving therapy: A social competence approach to clinical intervention*. New York: Springer.

Ellis, A. (1989). Rational-emotive therapy. In R. J. Corsini & D. Wedding (Eds.), *Current psychotherapies* (pp. 197–240). Itasca, IL: Peacock.

Ellis, A., & Dryden, W. (2007). *The practice of rational emotive behavior therapy* (2nd ed.). New York: Springer.

Falloon, I. R., Boyd, J. L., & McGill, C. (1984). Problem-solving training. In *Family care of schizophrenia* (pp. 261–284). New York: Guilford Press.

Foa, E., Hembree, E., & Rothbaum, B. O. (2007). *Prolonged exposure therapy for PTSD: Emotional processing of traumatic experiences: Therapist guide*. New York: Oxford University Press.

Foa, E., Yadin, E., & Lichner, T. K. (2012). *Exposure and response (ritual) prevention for obsessive–compulsive disorder: Therapist guide* (2nd ed.). New York: Oxford University Press.

Fox, E., Mathews, A., Calder, A. J., & Yiend, J. (2007). Anxiety and sensitivity to gaze direction in emotionally expressive faces. *Emotion, 7*, 478–486.

Gaillot, M. T., & Baumeister, R. F. (2007). The physiology of willpower: Linking blood glucose to self-control. *Personality and Social Psychology Review, 11*, 303–327.

Gilbert, P., & Leahy, R. L. (2007). *The therapeutic relationship in the cognitive behavioral psychotherapies*. London: Routledge.

Gottman, J. M., & Katz, L. F. (1990). Effects of marital discord on young children's peer interaction and health. *Developmental Psychology, 25*, 373–381.

Gratz, K. L., Rosenthal, M. Z., Tull, M. T., Lejuez, C. W., & Gunderson, J. G. (2006). An experimental investigation of emotion dysregulation in borderline personality disorder. *Journal of Abnormal Psychology, 115*, 850–855.

Gross, J. J., & Thompson, R. A. (2009). Emotion regulation: Conceptual foundations. In J. J. Gross (Ed.), *Handbook of emotion regulation* (pp. 3–24). New York: Guilford Press.

Harmon-Jones, E., & Peterson, C. K. (2009). Supine body position reduces neural response to anger evocation. *Psychological Science, 20*, 1209–1210.

Harned, M. S., Korslund, K. E., & Linehan, M. M. (2014). A pilot randomized controlled trial of dialectical behavior therapy with and without the dialectical behavior therapy prolonged exposure protocol for suicidal and self-injuring women with borderline personality disorder and PTSD. *Behaviour Research and Therapy, 55*, 7–17.

Hawton, K., & Kirk, J. (1989). Problem-solving. In K. Hawton, P. M. Salvkovskis, J. Kirk, & D. M. Clark (Eds.), *Cognitive behavior therapy for psychiatric problems: A practical guide* (pp. 406–426). Oxford, UK: Oxford University Press.

Heard, H. L. (2002). Psychotherapeutic approaches to suicidal ideation and behaviour. In K. Hawton & K. van Heeringen (Eds.), *The international handbook of suicide and attempted suicide* (pp. 503–518). Chichester, West Sussex, UK: Wiley.

Heard, H. L., & Linehan, M. M. (1993). Problems of self and borderline personality disorder: A dialectical behavioral analysis. In Z. V. Segal & S. J. Blatt (Eds.), *The self in emotional distress: Cognitive and psychodynamic perspectives* (pp. 301–325). New York: Guilford Press.

Heard, H. L., & Linehan, M. M. (1994, November). The volatile and relational self clusters in borderline personality disorder. In R. M. Turner (Chair), *The empirical identification of subgroups of borderline personality disorder patients*. Symposium conducted at the meeting of the Association for Advancement of Behavior Therapy, San Diego, CA.

Heard, H. L., & Linehan, M. M. (2005). Integrative therapy for borderline personality disorder. In J. C. Norcross & M. R. Goldfried (Eds.), *Handbook of psychotherapy integration* (pp. 299–320). New York: Oxford University Press.

Jamieson, J. P., Mendes, W. B., & Nock, M. K. (2013). Improving acute stress responses: The power of reappraisal. *Current Directions in Psychological Science, 22*, 51–56.

Jones, M. C. (1924). The elimination of children's fears. *Journal of Experimental Psychology, 7*, 383–390.

Kabat-Zinn, J. (1994). *Wherever you go there you are: Mindfulness meditation in everyday life*. New York: Hyperion.

Kashdan, T. B., Ferssizidis, P., Collins, R. L., & Muraven, M. (2010). Emotion differentiation as resilience against excessive alcohol use: An ecological momentary assessment in underage social drinkers. *Psychological Science, 21*, 1341–1347.

Kashdan, T. B., & Rottenberg, J. (2010). Psychological flexibility as a fundamental aspect of health. *Clinical Psychology Review, 30*, 865–878.

Kegan, R. (1982). *The evolving self: Problem and process in human development*. Cambridge, MA: Harvard University Press.

Klonsky, E. D. (2007). The functions of deliberate self-injury: A review of the evidence. *Clinical Psychology Review, 27*, 226–239.

Leible, T. L., & Snell, W. E., Jr. (2004). Borderline personality disorder and multiple aspects of emotional intelligence. *Personality and Individual Differences, 37*, 393–404.

Leotti, L. A., & Delgado, M. R. (2011). The inherent reward of choice. *Psychological Science, 22*, 1310–1318.

Leotti, L. A., Iyengar, S. S., & Ochsner, K. N. (2010). Born to choose: The origins and value of the need for control. *Trends in Cognitive Sciences, 14*, 457–463.

Levine, D., Marziali, E., & Hood, J. (1997). Emotion processing in borderline personality disorders. *Journal of Nervous and Mental Disease, 185*, 240–246.

Levins, R., & Lewontin, R. (1985). *The dialectical biologist*. Cambridge, MA: Harvard University Press.

Lieberman, M. D., Eisenberger, N. I., Crockett, M. J., Tom, S. M., Pfeifer, J. H., & Way, B. M. (2007). Putting feelings into words: Affect labeling disrupts amygdala activity in response to affective stimuli. *Psychological Science, 18*, 421–428.

Linehan, M. M. (1993a). *Cognitive-behavioral treatment of borderline personality disorder*. New York: Guilford Press.

Linehan, M. M. (1993b). *Skills training manual for treating borderline personality disorder*. New York: Guilford Press.

Linehan, M. M. (1997). Validation and psychotherapy. In A. Bohart & L. Greenberg (Eds.), *Empathy reconsidered: New directions in psychotherapy* (pp. 353–392). Washington, DC: American Psychological Association.

Linehan, M. M. (2014). *DBT skills training manual* (2nd ed.). New York: Guilford Press.

Linehan, M. M., & Heard, H. L. (1993). Impact of treatment accessibility on clinical course of parasuicidal patients: In reply to R. E. Hoffman [Letter to the editor]. *Archives of General Psychiatry, 50*, 157–158.

Linehan, M. M., & Schmidt, H., III. (1995). The dialectics of effective treatment of borderline personality disorder. In W. O'Donoghue & L. Krasner (Eds.), *Theories in behavior therapy: Exploring behavior change* (pp. 553–584). Washington, DC: American Psychological Association.

Linehan, M. M., Tutek, D. A., Heard, H. L., & Armstrong, H. E. (1994). Interpersonal outcomes of cognitive behavioral treatment for chronically suicidal borderline patients. *American Journal of Psychiatry, 151*, 1771–1776.

Longe, S. E., Wise, R., Bantick, S., Lloyd, D., Johansen-Berg, H., McGlone, F., et al. (2001). Counter-stimulatory effects on pain perception and processing are significantly altered by attention: An fMRI study. *NeuroReport, 12*, 2021–2025.

McLeavey, B. C., Daly, R. J., Ludgate, J. W., & Murray, C. M. (1994) Interpersonal problem solving skills training in the treatment of self-poisoning patients. *Suicide and Life Threatening Behavior, 24*, 382–394.

McRae, K., Hughes, B., Chopra, S., Gabrieli, J. D., Gross, J. J., & Ochsner, K. N. (2010). The neural bases of distraction and reappraisal. *Journal of Cognitive Neuroscience, 22,* 248–262.

Meichenbaum, D., & Turk, D. (1987). *Facilitating treatment adherence: A practitioner's guidebook.* New York: Plenum.

Miller, A. L., Rathus, J. H., & Linehan, M. L. (2006). *Dialectical behavior therapy with suicidal adolescents.* New York: Guilford Press.

Morin, C. M., Bootzin, R. R., Buysse, D. J., Edinger, J. D., Collin, A., Espie, C. A., et al. (2006). Psychological and behavioral treatment of insomnia: Update of the recent evidence (1998–2004). *Sleep, 29,* 1398–1413.

Morin, C. M., Hauri, P. J., Espie, C. A., Spielman, A. J., Buysse, D. J., & Bootzin, R. R. (1999). Nonpharmacologic treatment of chronic insomnia: An American Academy of Sleep Medicine review. *Sleep, 22,* 1134–1156.

Neacsiu, A. D., Rizvi, S. L., & Linehan, M. M. (2010). Dialectical behavior therapy skills use as a mediator and outcome of treatment for borderline personality disorder. *Behaviour Research and Therapy, 48,* 832–839.

Nezu, A. M., Nezu, C. M., & Perri, M. G. (1989). *Problem-solving therapy for depression: Theory, research and clinical guidelines.* New York: Wiley.

Nock, M. K., & Prinstein, M. J. (2004). A functional approach to the assessment of self-mutilative behavior. *Journal of Consulting and Clinical Psychology, 75,* 885–890.

Pavlov, I. P. (1927). *Conditioned reflexes: An investigation of the physiological activity of the cerebral cortex.* New York: Oxford University Press.

Plato. (1969). *The last days of Socrates* (3rd ed., H. Tredennick, Trans.). New York: Penguin Books.

Reps, P., & Senzaki, N. (1985). *Zen flesh, Zen bones.* Rutland, VT: Tuttle.

Rizvi, S. L., & Linehan, M. M. (2005). The treatment of maladaptive shame in borderline personality disorder: A pilot study of "opposite action." *Cognitive and Behavioral Practice, 12,* 437–447.

Rode, S., Salkovskis, P. M., & Jack, T. (2001). An experimental study of attention, labeling and memory in people suffering from chronic pain. *Pain, 94,* 193–203.

Rosenthal, T. L., & Bandura, A. (1978). Psychological modeling: Theory and practice. In S. L. Garfield & A. E. Bergin (Eds.), *Handbook of psychotherapy and behavior change* (2nd ed., pp. 621–658). New York: Wiley.

Safer, D., Robinson, A., & Jo, B. (2010). Outcome from a randomized controlled trial of group therapy for binge eating disorder: Comparing dialectical behavior therapy adapted for binge eating to an active comparison group therapy. *Behavior Therapy, 41,* 106–120.

Safer, D. L., Telch, C. F., & Agras, W. S. (2001). Dialectical behavior therapy for bulimia nervosa. *American Journal of Psychiatry, 58,* 632–634.

Salkovskis, P. M., Atha, C., & Storer, D. (1990) Cognitive-behavioral problem solving in the treatment of patients who repeatedly attempt suicide: A controlled trial. *British Journal of Psychiatry, 157,* 871–876.

Schumacher, J. E., Milby, J. B., Wallace, D., Meehan, D. C., Kertesz, S., Vuchinich, R., et al. (2007). Meta-analysis of day treatment and contingency-management dismantling research: Birmingham Homeless Cocaine

Studies (1990–2006). *Journal of Consulting and Clinical Psychology, 75,* 823–828.

Sheppes, G., & Meiran, N. (2007). Better late than never?: On the dynamics of on-line regulation of sadness using distraction and cognitive reappraisal. *Personality and Social Psychology Bulletin, 33,* 1518–1532.

Skinner, B. F. (1953). *Science and human behavior.* New York: Macmillan.

Skinner, B. F. (1976). *About behaviorism.* New York: Random House.

Soler, J., Valdeperez, A., Feliu-Soler, A., Pascual, J. C., Portella, M. J., Martin-Blanco, A., et al. (2011). Effects of the dialectical behavioral therapy mindfulness module on attention in patients with borderline personality disorder. *Behavioral Research and Therapy, 50,* 150–157.

Staats, A. W. (1975). *Social behaviorism.* Homewood, IL: Dorsey Press.

Swann, W. B., Stein-Seroussi, A., & Giesler, R. B. (1992). Why people self-verify. *Journal of Personality and Social Psychology, 62,* 392–401.

Telch, C. F., Agras, W. S., & Linehan, M. M. (2001). Dialectical behavior therapy for binge eating disorder. *Journal of Consulting and Clinical Psychology, 69,* 1061–1065.

Thiruchselvam, R., Blechert, J., Sheppes, G., Rydstrom, A., & Gross, J. J. (2011). The temporal dynamics of emotion regulation: An EEG study of distraction and reappraisal. *Biological Psychology, 87,* 84–92.

Thiruchselvam, R., Hajcak, G., & Gross, J. J. (2012). Looking inward: Shifting attention within working memory representations alters emotional responses. *Psychological Science, 23,* 1461–1466.

Trupin, E. W., Stewart, D. G., Beach, B., & Boesky, L. (2002). Effectiveness of a dialectical behavior therapy program for incarcerated female juvenile offenders. *Child and Adolescent Mental Health, 7,* 121–127.

Tucker, R. C. (Ed.). (1978). *The Marx–Engels reader* (2nd ed.). New York: Norton.

Van der Sande, R., van Rooijen, E., Buskens, E., Allart, E., Hawton, K., van der Graaf, Y., et al. (1997). Intensive in-patient and community intervention versus routine care after attempted suicide: A randomized controlled intervention. *British Journal of Psychiatry, 171,* 35–41.

Watson, J. B., & Rayner, R. (1920). Conditioned emotional reactions. *Journal of Experimental Psychology, 3,* 1–14.

Webster's new collegiate dictionary. (1981). New York: World Publishing.

Westphal, M., Seivert, N. H., & Bonanno, G. A. (2010). Expressive flexibility. *Emotion, 10,* 92–100.

Williams, J. M. G., & Swales, M. A. (2004). The use of mindfulness-based approaches for suicidal patients. *Archives of Suicide Research, 8*(4), 315–329.

Wilson, G. T., & O'Leary, K. D. (1980). *Principles of behavior therapy.* Englewood Cliffs, NJ: Prentice-Hall.

Wolpe, J. (1958). *Psychotherapy by reciprocal inhibition.* Stanford, CA: Stanford University Press.

INDEX

Note: *f* or *t* following a page number indicates a figure or a table.